Managing Mental Health Services

Health Services Management

Series Editors:
Chris Ham, Health Services Management Centre, University of Birmingham
Chris Heginbotham, Chief Executive, East and North Hertfordshire Health
Authority

The British National Health Service is one of the biggest and most complex organisations in the developed world. Employing around one million people and involving high levels of public expenditure, the Service is of major concern to both the public and politicians. Management within the NHS faces a series of challenges in ensuring that resources are deployed efficiently and effectively. These challenges include the planning and management of human resources, the integration of professionals into the management process, and making sure that services meet the needs of patients and the public.

Against this background, the Health Services Management series addresses the many issues and practical problems faced by people in managerial roles in health services.

Managing Mental Health Services

*Amanda Reynolds
and Graham Thornicroft*

Open University Press
Buckingham · Philadelphia

Open University Press
Celtic Court
22 Ballmoor
Buckingham
MK18 1XW

email: enquiries@openup.co.uk
world wide web: www.openup.co.uk

and
325 Chestnut Street
Philadelphia, PA 19106, USA

First Published 1999
Reprinted 2000, 2001

ISBN 0 335 19834 1 (hb)   0 335 19833 3 (pb)

A catalogue record of this book is available from the British Library

Library of Congress Cataloging-in-Publication Data
Reynolds, Amanda, 1967–
    Managing mental health services / Amanda Reynolds and Graham Thornicrof
      p. cm. – (Health services management)
    Includes bibliographical references and index.
    ISBN 0–335–19833–3. — ISBN 0–335–19834–1
    1. Mental health services—Administration. I. Title. II. Series.
  RA790.5.R5 1999
  362.2'068—dc21
                                     98–30735
                                         CIP

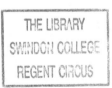
Copy-edited and typeset by The Running Head Limited, Cambridge

Printed and bound in Great Britain by
Marston Lindsay Ross International Ltd,
Oxfordshire

Contents

Acknowledgements

We are very pleased to acknowledge the many colleagues who have made direct or indirect contributions to this book. We have been inspired in particular by Douglas Bennett, Jim Birley, Bill Breakey, Lorenzo Burti, Eric Byers, David Clark, Julie Craig, Geoff Doodson, Barbara Epps, Jane Field, Michol Fisher, Juliana Fredrick, Gyles Glover, David Goldberg, Helen Hally, Bernadette Hennigan, Frank Holloway, Paul James, Rachel Jenkins, Paul Lelliot, Jan McHugh, Barbara Morris, Steven Morris, Derek Nicoll, Malcolm Philip, Sally Pitts-Brown, Alan Rosen, Geoff Shepherd, Dave Shiress, Geraldine Strathdee, George Szmukler, Michele Tansella, Paul Ward and Estella Weston. We are pleased to acknowledge *Private Eye* for allowing us to reproduce the cartoons in this book. We have been grateful throughout the writing of this book for the continuing support of Jacinta Evans at the Open University Press, and her patience on more than one occasion! In addition, we have benefited from superb commentary on this book by Pat Earing and Patrick Creehan.

Section A
Context

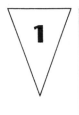

1 Introduction

Mental health services are important, complex and changing fast. They are important because mental disorders affect a quarter of all adults each year, and specialist services consume about 12 per cent of the National Health Service (NHS) budget. They are complex because they require the close collaboration of many specialities and agencies to help service users most effectively. They remain in rapid transition, since a third of the large asylums have closed, a further third are now in the process of decommissioning, and new policies and laws continue to rain down upon all of us.

In this book we shall draw upon our own experience of developing community mental health services in South London in recent years. As we carried out a substantial change agenda in a relatively short period of time we became aware of how difficult it is to bring about and sustain service improvement. As our own service transition gained pace, recurrent themes emerged. We became aware of the need to provide staff at all levels of the service with a clear direction, and to convey a satisfactory justification of the changes. We also recognized the many different routes that individuals take as they develop management responsibilities. Staff have different types and levels of training, experience and expectations of the management role. People who find themselves in NHS management come from many backgrounds: nursing, medical and allied professions, NHS administration, other public service organizations, and from the private sector. To respond to this diversity we have split this book into two clear and separate sections. These two sections are *Six key steps for developing manageable mental health services* and *The six key managerial tasks*. Our primary aim is to convey a whole-system managerial view of mental health services.

This is a book about organizational survival for both individuals and services. It is a book about the real situations that a manager encounters in mental health service delivery. To succeed in the present-day National Health Service managers must deploy staff, resources and their own time effectively. Clinicians also need to react appropriately and be proactive to function effectively in their organization. They find themselves increasingly measured by their service activity, quality and the evidence-base for their particular services or treatments. We shall therefore seek to give practical insights and realistic tips on dealing with many of these pressures.

This book will help managers to understand the mental health service environment, and to adapt and develop effective services to meet the needs of their local population. Some readers of this book will be new to management roles and will need a quick A–Z reference to the key issues. Other readers will have been in the service longer and will need an update to allow them to take a fresh approach. For both groups, our aim is to help you to make your organization work better for service users. We offer suggestions on spotting staff in trouble and teams that are dysfunctional, so that you can harness individual and team strengths. Through this approach we want to encourage you in the development of high quality, sustainable services. As you understand more of the context of the organization you work in, we expect that your own role can become more fulfilling and you may be better able to understand the contributions of other agencies. We want to encourage collaboration, rather than the isolation that many of us have encountered in the past.

One of the main goals of this book is to break down large complex tasks and change agendas into small achievable steps and goals. We have found that when tasks are systematically broken down, their vastness can be managed within realistic timescales, and people feel more motivated to participate. Throughout the book we shall relate the material and themes to current challenges in the National Health Service, which include:

- the importance of, and benefits of, joint working between clinicians and management
- the relevance of evidence-based medicine to clinical practice in mental health services
- the growing move towards the use of research evidence in the purchasing of mental health services
- the need to relate the local provision of services to national trends
- the importance of getting individuals and teams working effectively.

We have recent experience from the 'coalface' of the barriers to managing community mental health services. We are therefore not speaking to you from within a business school or from a training department. All the ideas and principles that we describe in this book are drawn from our own experience, some of which were successful, and some unsuccessful. We have also described some of these failed attempts, and it may be useful for you to see what we tried, why it did not work, and what alternatives we would now consider. For us the intrinsic challenge in service management is how to move from ideas to practice. The book therefore seeks to be practical, pragmatic and opportunistic. It is about real services and often, therefore, about managing in a messy world.

Each chapter will include an overview of the relevant background literature, and the format will include lists of key points. We shall illustrate the practice and learning points with examples taken directly from our own service experience. We expect that you are busy, and so we have designed the book so that it can be used in different ways. Readers can work through chapter by chapter, or dip in and out of the various sections. It can be used for formal training on management courses or, more informally, the chapters can be read and discussed in the office.

Our focus on real-life case studies and situations will demonstrate the achievability of major change within a health care setting. The emphasis will be on staff as the key resource and on how to utilize their strengths to obtain the best treatment and care for service users. We shall encourage you to develop and change services, and also to consider the impact of change and change programmes on staff and service users themselves. We shall also describe the importance of preserving what is already effective in your service.

Each chapter will build on the previous as we seek to guide you through a six-step process of service development:

Step 1   The vision: agreeing the guiding principles
Step 2   Estimating population needs
Step 3   Making an organizational diagnosis
Step 4   Writing the strategic service plan
Step 5   Delivering the service components
Step 6   Review and evaluation.

This book is written so that it is clearly understandable by the range of middle management and senior clinical staff who are often called upon to implement community mental health policies, but who may not have a detailed background training in change management, service planning, epidemiology, health service research, or in project management!

We begin this discussion in Chapter 2 by putting our ideas into the context of national and government policy on mental health provision. Managers are now frequently asked to respond to local levels of *need for services*; they see this as an onerous and complex task. In Chapter 3 we shall guide readers through basic values, and through ways to establish levels of local need for services in Chapter 4. There we summarize some of the latest measures available for assessing mental health need locally, and how to establish the types of services likely to be required.

As a way of putting all of these ideas into context we advise readers to make an organizational and team diagnosis, which we outline in Chapter 5. This is a means of establishing the current functioning of the service, examining its strengths and areas of weakness along with identifying potential blocks to change. We intend to guide you towards making a systematic view of the current organizational health of where you work. Then we go on to describe the detailed work of writing the *strategic business plan* in Chapter 6, which is a concise statement of where the service is now, where you want it to move to, and how to get there. It is also important to outline in detail *the service components* that will need to be provided, and we do this in Chapter 7, along with a consideration of the many clinical and managerial interfaces between the service components. Chapter 8 gives an overview of how services can be monitored and evaluated to assess whether they are performing according to plan.

Among other aims, this book will also seek to demystify management and to outline the key principles for all involved in service management to consider and practise. Often management has been seen by clinicians as something vague, or about grey-suited graduates sitting in offices writing mission statements! We shall proceed by breaking down the management role into six key tasks, which are described in Chapters 9 to 14:

Task 1 Managing the change process
Task 2 The central role of human resources
Task 3 Managing budgets
Task 4 Creating a robust infrastructure
Task 5 Allies or adversaries? (*with Dr Richard Byng and Sally Pitts-Brown*)
Task 6 Managing the future.

We intend that our discussion of these six key managerial tasks will help to round out your skills and fill any gaps in your previous training or experience. This may relate to how to make budgets work for you, which we précis in Chapter 11. Budgets and budget management can be a complex task, so we shall try to simplify the jargon and show you the enjoyable side of devolved budget management, by helping you to remain one step ahead of the game. One key function of effective management is the coordination and release of individual potential within teams, and the consequent improvement in services and systems. In managing the staff and maximizing their potential we offer examples of recruitment, objective setting, and ways of reviewing staff and team performance.

Management in the NHS often feels rushed, as people are frequently managing large and diverse professional groups alongside other competing demands. It is common to get bogged down in the day-to-day detail and to work only by relating to outside events. We shall suggest ways to develop a less crowded perspective of management and on how to protect proactive thinking and planning time for yourself and your staff.

None of this can be done alone, and in Chapter 13 we describe the importance of seeing the manager's role as one of a series of partnerships with tactical and strategic allies. We reflect on our own lessons in the challenges of setting up community-orientated services – working with neighbours, for example, and with the fear that mental illness can often generate locally. We also look at how to encourage the participation of service users in the planning, management and delivery of local services. We then consider how to ensure the support of those more senior in your organization, whether commissioner or provider, in key initiatives in joint commissioning of services between health, housing, social services and the voluntary sector. A book addressing the key managerial tasks for mental health services also needs to explore the issues relating to the planning and providing of services, and these are addressed in Chapter 14.

The book is a distillation of policies, research, and managerial and clinical experience in relation to mental health services. In many areas these services are moving quickly away from immobility (in terms of the quality of service offered until recently in many larger asylums) towards a decentralized and constantly shifting array of service segments. The challenge is to keep a picture of the whole service system in mind, and to implement the service components in a way that does not produce fragmentation in practice. In *Managing Mental Health Services* we want to help those managing mental health services to learn quickly from the experience of others, and to have access to the best available information on how to guide services for the benefit of the service users we serve.

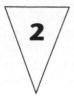

2 Policy background

Key themes

In this chapter we aim to:

- bring you up to date on the current range of policy requirements
- clarify the confusing jargon used in these government documents
- help you see the guidance as an opportunity to build upon good clinical and managerial practice
- identify the Care Programme Approach as the cornerstone for adult mental illness service delivery
- explain more recent measures including the Supervision Register and Supervised Discharge
- enable you to be aware of and act on the recommendations from the major inquiries.

Introduction

What are the basic building blocks of government policy and guidance for mental health services? Here we present a brief overview of the many recent and important policy and legal changes you need to be familiar with (Table 2.1). These policies now form the framework of law and guidance for our managerial work. We realize that these policies have been introduced rapidly and in large numbers; many managers are not yet fully aware of these basic policy-building blocks, and the way they affect the services we are expected to deliver. Yet some policies or sets of guidance are not fully operational in all areas, and as Peck and colleagues say in the King's Fund

Table 2.1   Key reports in the development of community care policy

1988	Report by Sir Roy Griffiths: *Community Care: An Agenda for Action*
1990	National Health Service and Community Care Act
1990	Department of Health guidance, 'Care Programme Approach'
1994	Department of Health, *Health of the Nation, Key Area Handbook, Mental Illness*
1994	Introduction of supervision registers
1995	Zito Trust report, *Learning the Lessons* (Shepherd 1996)
1996	Mental Health (Patients in the Community) Act
1996	*Spectrum of Care* (NHS Executive 1996a)

London Commission Mental Health Report, 'It is reasonable to assume that implementation of particular policy requirements will take longer than policy makers may wish' Peck *et al.* (1997: 347). Knowing the details of these policies will help you: (i) to make decisions that are consistent with national policy, (ii) allow you to talk to your local planners in a shared language, (iii) have realistic expectations of the roles of other agencies, (iv) prioritize your time to work mainly on projects that harmonize with the overall goals set by the NHS Executive, and (v) meet the demands set on you by contracts, recommendations from mental health inquiries reports and from central government.

In this chapter we summarize the main components of current policy on services for adults who suffer from mental illnesses, which include: (i) the 1988 Griffiths Report, (ii) the NHS and Community Care Act 1990, (iii) the 1990 Care Programme Approach, (iv) the 1994 *Health of the Nation* report, (v) the 1994 Ritchie Report into the care and treatment of Christopher Clunis, (vi) the House of Commons Health Select Committee Report 1994, (vii) the 1994 supervision register, (viii) the 1996 proposals of the Mental Health (Patients in the Community) Act, which introduced Supervised Discharge Orders, (ix) the *Spectrum of Care* proposals 1996, and (x) the 1996 report on 24-hour nursed care.

The NHS and Community Care Act 1990

The NHS and Community Care Act was passed in 1990, aiming to bring greater coordination to the provision of community care by the health and social services. In essence it introduced the following important changes: a distinction between purchasing and providing functions, the requirement for local community care plans, the creation of provider trusts and fundholding general practices, and the transfer of funds for residential care from the Department of Social Security to the social services, which was effective from 1 April 1993. Because this Act has such widespread and fundamental influences upon the NHS and upon local authorities, we shall focus here upon its central implications for mental health managers. The objectives of the NHS and Community Care Act 1990 are:

- to promote the development of domiciliary, day and respite services to enable people to live in their own homes wherever feasible and sensible
- to promote the development of a flourishing independent sector alongside good quality public services
- to coordinate social care by the 'care manager'
- to make proper assessments of need
- to provide services on the basis of needs assessments, to clarify the responsibilities of agencies and so make it easier to hold them to account for their performance
- to secure better value for taxpayers' money by introducing a new funding structure for social care
- to ensure that service providers make practical support for carers a high priority.

The Act reinforced the already established need to produce annually a local *community care plan* to go to the NHS Executive with details of the mental health service for the following year and beyond. It needs to be agreed by the chief officer of the local health and social service provider agencies, and to be formally endorsed by the local health authority and by elected members of the social services committee. This plan sets the framework within which more detailed local plans are developed and funded. At the local level, health and social services have established joint planning teams or joint community care planning groups, whose functions include writing an annual community care plan and bidding for mental illness-specific grants and other government allocations. These are strategic forums that oversee inter-agency initiatives and play a part in prioritizing local projects for funding.

A key role that has been defined in the Act is that of the *care manager*. 'Care management' needs a special word of clarification. The term was introduced in 1991 as a variation of the term 'case manager', which had been used for the previous decade in the USA. 'Care manager' describes the role of qualified social workers, who assess the needs of service users and who then purchase direct care services from other providers. It is different from the role of health service 'key workers', who assess needs and who then also provide direct care. The Act makes the following statutory requirements of care managers:

> where it appears to a local authority that any person for whom they may provide or arrange for the provision of community care services may be in need of any such services, the authority (a) shall carry out an assessment of his needs for those services and (b) having regard to the results of that assessment, shall then decide whether his needs call for the provision by them of any such services.
>
> (NHS and Community Care Act 1990)

The assessment of need by both social and health services is a requirement of the Care Programme Approach. Social services are also required under the NHS and Community Care Act 1990 to provide an assessment of social care needs to all those who require one, including those with mental disorder, and these types of assessment should overlap as much as is practicable.

A central part of the guidance associated with the Act concerns *needs assessment*. Needs can be defined on a population or individual basis, and from the perspectives of politicians, clinicians, carers and service users; clearly these will differ. A working definition of need in the sense in which it is used in the Care Programme Approach is that a need exists where the service user 'is able in some way to benefit from care', whether this care is medical or social. The needs are not limited to the care that happens to be available; a broader definition of need may suggest services that should be developed.

It is important to recognize that the purchaser–provider divisions (which have been established within both the health and social services authorities) occur at different levels. Within social services departments, 'purchasing' is much more orientated to the individual, whereas within the NHS it is orientated to entire service systems. In so far as this affects care management arrangements, it is less critical where social services are the main purchaser of services, for example in provision for people with learning disabilities. It is however of much greater importance where the health authority is the main purchaser of community services, for example mental health. In such cases, the work of the individual care manager will require considerable support by local NHS provider services.

The Care Programme Approach

The Care Programme Approach (CPA) is a measure the government instructed mental health and social services to introduce in 1991 (Department of Health 1990). It consists of the development of personalized care packages for all patients accepted by the specialist psychiatric services, to ensure that they receive the care they need. It aims to guide good clinical practice, and to prevent service users from 'slipping through the net' of follow-up. The CPA is a central part of the government's mental health policy, and was brought in following concern that, after discharge, many service users did not have a named member of staff to contact, nor was there a defined care plan. The CPA (Department of Health 1990) consists of four parts, namely:

Assessment of health and social care needs

The systematic assessment of needs begins with a good clinical and social history that covers both the needs for diagnosis and treatment, and needs for social care. Most service users with severe mental illnesses will have a wide range of needs, and a full assessment will involve information from informants: family, friends, professional and non-professional carers.

Social workers, who have parallel assessment and 'care management' procedures, should be involved in more complex assessments, and these may be carried out jointly. A full needs assessment may require a multi-disciplinary meeting. Risk of self-harm, self-neglect, or harm to others, should be assessed.

Written care plan

For in-patients, or out-patients who need multi-disciplinary input, a care plan should be agreed at a ward round or CPA meeting, with everyone who will be involved in implementing it. The plan should be agreed as far as possible with the service user, and with carers. For other service users, this might simply involve a plan for out-patient treatment being written in the notes after completing a history and examination, though even this should be discussed and agreed with the service user.

Key worker

The key worker has responsibility for the coordination of the care programme. If the service user moves to another area, a proper handover should be made by the key worker to another team. The key worker should be the professional with the closest relationship with the service user; this will often be a community psychiatric nurse (CPN) or social worker, but could be a psychiatrist in training. Each key worker will usually need to nominate a 'deputy' for periods of sickness or planned leave.

Regular reviews

The care plan should usually be reviewed at least every six months, but the key worker should be able to arrange for a review meeting with others involved in the service user's care if the care plan is not being effectively carried out. A register of names of service users needing reviews should be kept ('CPA register'), and reminders of the need for review issued. There are important implications of this system of reviews for shared documentation of care plan and CPA reviews, and for the supporting information systems.

The Care Programme Approach in practice

Who should receive the Care Programme Approach? The CPA applies to all service users under the care of specialist psychiatric services. However, not every service user can or should have multi-disciplinary team reviews. The CPA can be 'tiered', with most service users needing a 'minimal' CPA in which the basic elements of the CPA are represented by a written care plan in the notes, and the out-patient doctor, general practitioner or CPN acting as key worker and coordinating the follow-up. For other cases, an intermediate level of CPA can be applied, perhaps with brief reviews at team meetings or discussions between the staff involved; only more complex cases will require regular full multi-disciplinary review meetings.

There are important implications within the CPA for communication and confidentiality. The care plan will often involve non-NHS bodies, e.g. voluntary sector housing, and good communication with them about the care plan is essential. However, the care plan is a medical record and the service user's right to confidentiality must be respected. Permission should be sought before communicating information beyond the professionals involved, and if this is not given, confidentiality can only be breached in exceptional circumstances in the public interest, a decision that must be made by the consultant. This may be a particular issue in relation to the sharing of client information between health and social services.

In terms of the timing of the CPA in relation to discharge from hospital, a CPA meeting should take place before discharge to ensure that the necessary community services will be in place. In the case of detained service users, this can also serve as a 'section 117' meeting, where the aftercare required by section 117 of the Mental Health Act 1983 is planned. If an adequate care plan cannot be put into practice, the service user should not be discharged.

The 1995 NHS Executive document *Building Bridges* set out a revised, tiered approach to implementing the CPA (Department of Health 1995). The tiers of the Care Programme Approach are:

Minimal CPA
- limited health care needs
- low support needs
- stable illness
- usually one practitioner involved.

More complex CPA
- medium level of support needed
- often more than one service involved
- needs less likely to remain stable
- require multi-disciplinary assessments
- allocate a key worker.

Full multi-disciplinary CPA
- for people with severe mental illness and severe social dysfunction or who present significant risk
- allocate key worker
- consider inclusion on supervision register.

The importance of the Care Programme Approach

The CPA represents a managed process of care that remains as the cornerstone for all other aspects of policy for services for the adult severely mentally ill. The limitations of the CPA also need to be recognized, as it does not in itself contribute anything to direct face-to-face treatment and support. There remain considerable local variations in how far the CPA has been implemented. The CPA requires considerable effort initially to establish the appropriate administrative system, so can this expense be justified in terms of improved service user care? The importance of the CPA is that it is designed to target resources on those who need them most, to ensure that vulnerable people continue to receive the care they need, and to coordinate the delivery of such care.

The Health of the Nation

Mental health was included as one of five 'key areas' of the five-year national health strategy set out in the 1992 framework *The Health of the Nation* (Department of Health 1993). The first target has led directly to the creation of the *Health of the Nation* Outcomes Scale (HoNOS), and the use in future of the scale and the inclusion of the suicide targets are likely to feature increasingly in purchaser–provider contracts (Wing *et al.* 1998). The *Health of the Nation* mental health targets were:

- to improve significantly the health and social functioning of mentally ill people
- to reduce the overall suicide rate by at least 15 per cent by the year 2000 (from 11.1 per 100,000 population in 1990 to no more than 9.4)
- to reduce the suicide rate of severely mentally ill people by at least 33 per cent by the year 2000 (from the estimate of 15 per cent in 1990 to no more than 10 per cent).

The supervision register

The supervision register (SR) is an administrative measure the government instructed mental health services to introduce in 1994 (NHS Executive 1994b). It was felt to be necessary because of concerns, such as those expressed in the report of the Inquiry into the Care of Christopher Clunis, that the CPA was not being provided for service users 'who may be at greatest risk and need most support'. The SR is intended to apply to a small group of service users who already fall into the 'full multi-disciplinary' tier of the CPA, and in practice may be regarded as the most intensive tier of the CPA. The supervision register applies to those 'known to be at significant risk or potentially at significant risk of committing serious violence, or suicide or of serious self-neglect as the result of severe and enduring mental illness' (NHS Executive 1994b), and requires allocation of a key worker and a risk assessment.

It is a list of names, 'held locally by each provider Trust', of patients with a severe mental illness who are known to be 'at significant risk', as defined above. The register should include the names of the service user, the

Responsible Medical Officer (RMO) and key worker, as well as the nature of the risk, and basic details of the CPA (date of registration, components of the care plan, and review date).

The service user should therefore be put on the supervision register if it is judged that there is a significant risk of serious violence, self-harm or self-neglect. Risk assessment is an inexact science, and the decision about what represents significant risk will be a matter of clinical judgement, usually in the context of multi-disciplinary team discussion, within agreed local procedures. The risk assessment may help decision making about suitable accommodation and supports on discharge, and assist appropriate confidential communication within and between agencies. It can also act as useful definition to help health and social services staff identify people at particular risk. In practice only a small proportion of service users on each team's caseload will be on the supervision register. This will allow resources to be prioritized for this group.

The 1995 Zito Trust report, *Learning the Lessons*

The 1995 report produced by the Zito Trust called *Learning the Lessons* (Shepherd 1996) summarizes the terms of reference and the recommendations of 36 inquiries into homicides involving the mentally ill which occurred between 1985 and 1996. It usefully organizes the recommendations under headings that include health services, social services, monitoring and inspection, GPs, and in-patient care. It provides essential and salutary reading for all mental health service managers and clinicians, and provides the best single source detailing the relevance of individual inquiries for all services (Peay 1998).

The Mental Health (Patients in the Community) Act 1995/ Supervised Discharge Orders

Supervised Discharge Orders (SDOs) were introduced by the Mental Health (Patients in the Community) Act 1995, which amends the Mental Health Act (for England) 1983. The Order complements, but is different from, the supervision register. It allows the Responsible Medical Officer (RMO) who is treating a service user under sections 3, 37, 47 or 48 of the Mental Health Act (MHA) to apply for powers of formal supervision of the service user after discharge from hospital, which will be exercised by a 'supervisor', typically a CPN acting as a key worker. The SDOs

- are an amendment to the Mental Health Act 1983
- allow legal supervision of service users after discharge
- require 'substantial risk' to or by the service user
- define 'supervision' as power to 'take or convey' the service user
- are similar to a Guardianship Order.

The application is made by the RMO to the provider unit managers. The service user must already have satisfied the conditions for detention under the MHA sections given above, and in addition, the RMO must believe that there will be a substantial risk of serious harm to the service user or to the safety of other people if the service user does not receive aftercare on discharge from hospital, and that the powers of supervised discharge are likely to help ensure that the service user receives aftercare, according to the CPA.

The application by the RMO must be supported by applications from another doctor approved under section 12(2), who could be the consultant providing community care ('Community RMO') if different from the RMO, or the GP, *and* from an approved social worker. The application must always include an agreed care plan.

The SDO only takes effect once the service user is both discharged from hospital and discharged from detention, so it does not apply while the service user is on leave of absence (section 17). The service user has a right of appeal to a Mental Health Review Tribunal. SDOs last for six months, and like section 3 the RMO can apply to renew it for six months, then for a year at a time. The service user can be required to reside in a particular place, to attend at set times for medical treatment, occupation, education or training, and the supervisor must be allowed access to the place of residence to see the service user. In these respects the legal powers are similar to those of a Guardianship Order.

The supervisor has the 'power to take and convey' the service user, to home or to a place of treatment, with police or ambulance support if necessary. This can only be done if it is likely to result in the service user then cooperating with treatment, as the supervisor cannot prevent the service user from leaving the place of treatment as soon as he/she arrives, and the service user cannot be forced to take treatment. If necessary, the service user could be assessed for detention in hospital under section 3.

Though the procedure is elaborate, the powers are limited, and cannot be used if they are ineffective, as they will be if the service user is determined not to cooperate with the care plan. They may restrict civil liberties without making it possible to deliver better care. There may be a small group of service users who are currently very difficult to care for who will respond to the more assertive treatment the supervisor can provide using an SDO. Since its recent introduction the SDO has so far been little used.

The 'Spectrum of Care'

Spectrum of Care was a booklet issued by the Department of Health in February 1996 (along with four other guidance documents), supplementing previous guidance given in the *Health of the Nation Key Area Handbook* (1994) and summarizing the components that should be offered to people with mental illness on a local level (see Table 2.2).

Table 2.2   Key components of the 'Spectrum of Care'

	Acute/emergency care	*Rehabilitation/ continuing care*
Home-based	• sector teams • sustainable out-of-hours cover • intensive home support	• domiciliary services • key workers • care management and Care Programme Approach
Day care	• day hospitals	• drop-in centres • support groups • employment groups • day care
Residential support	• crisis accommodation • acute units • local secure units	• ordinary housing • unstaffed group homes • adult placement schemes • residential care schemes • nursing homes • 24-hour nursed NHS accommodation • medium-secure units • high secure units

The 1996 NHS Executive report on 24-hour nursed care

Launched at the same time as the 'Spectrum of Care', the NHS Executive report on 24-hour nursed care focused on the needs of the 'new long stay' group (NHS Executive 1996c). Possibly numbering at least 5,000 in England and Wales, these people include many who respond only partially to acute treatment and who remain substantially disabled. They usually require transfer to longer-term high-intensity treatment and support, without which they often remain for too long in acute psychiatric beds. The NHS Executive report makes clear that when service users require facilities offering 24-hour nursing care, this is an NHS responsibility, as it was in the days when many more long-stay wards in psychiatric institutions were provided. 24-hour nursed care is for people with severe and enduring mental illness who need:

• daily mental state monitoring
• frequent monitoring of risk
• supervision of medication
• assistance with self-care and daily living
• support to access with day care/rehabilitation
• skilled management of challenging behaviour
• ongoing evening and weekend active support.

The likely client group for this service are people who are severely socially disabled by mental illness, and many similar service users in previous decades would have become long-term in-patients in psychiatric institutions. The development of these new services now requires in each local area a residential care strategy, which is carefully coordinated and costed by health and social service purchasers. The report also gives recommendations on the location, size, design, staffing and treatment appropriate for such settings. It makes clear that a local needs assessment exercise should be carried out by each health authority, followed by a strategy for the planned expansion of 24-hour nursed care. The central message of this document is *'whatever the ambiguities with other client groups, there should be no doubt that providing fully for this client group is an NHS responsibility'* (NHS Executive 1996c). Even so, managers in many areas will need to investigate how they can discharge this newly clarified responsibility within the available budgets.

Putting policy into practice

In writing this chapter we are reminded of the sheer volume of recent guidance, the rapid-fire nature of its release, and the confusing nature of the terminology used. Even so, the central difficulty faced in implementing reasonable care is the split often found in practice between the provisions of the Care Programme Approach and care management. In fact, the spirit behind both of these is almost identical. In each case the key worker/care manager has similar responsibilities. The core tasks of key worker/care manager are:

- designing the care package
- identifying patients (case finding)
- assessing needs
- coordinating service delivery
- monitoring service delivery
- evaluating the effectiveness of services
- modifying the care package
- repeating the cycle unless services no longer needed.

In practice the health care and social care needs assessments are often carried out and acted upon separately. Most elements of current policy at present are discretionary rather than obligatory. Local provider staff are therefore allowed some flexibility in implementing these forms of guidance in ways that are clinically realistic, locally relevant and closely shared between health and social services. At the same time, providers who are not acting in accordance with these policies will need to answer the question – when posed for example by purchasers and by regional mental health lead officers – why not. In addition to the Zito Trust report referred to earlier, a useful summary of the main lessons emerging from the inquiries has been prepared by Lelliot and colleagues and is given in Table 2.3.

Table 2.3 Key themes arising in inquiries into mental health services

Theme 1
Poor communication between agencies (7*); particularly between health and social services (5), between mental health services and housing departments (3) and between specialist mental health services and GPs (3). A related theme to this was that of poor joint working (4) which was at all levels from commissioning and strategy (2) to multi-disciplinary care delivery (3).

Theme 2
Problems with discharge from hospital (5). This particularly related to failure to follow section 117 procedures, assess need, develop an aftercare plan and communicate this adequately to other agencies.

Theme 3
Poor assessment of risk of violence (6). This emphasized particularly the need for better and more training in risk assessment (4) and the importance of disclosure of risk factors to those with a need to know.

Theme 4
Liaison with police and probation services (5). This related both to the involvement of police in receiving or providing information about people receiving care from mental health services (2) and the better involvement of mental health care workers in diversion from custody services (3).

Theme 5
Confidentiality and professional ethics (4). These were reported as barriers particularly between health and social services (2) and between mental health services and the police (2).

Theme 6
Adequacy and allocation of resources (9). The inadequacy of, or the need to protect, numbers of residential care places in London (including hospital beds) was a common theme (8). Specific mention was made of short-stay admission beds (4), medium-secure provision (4), and the importance of maintaining a wide range of community-based residential services (4) with Department of Health guidance on levels of provision. Comment was also made on the inadequacy of numbers of community workers (2) and of the provision of day care services (2). Allocation of resources was commented on both between competing groups, e.g. children, elderly, etc. (1), between health and social care (1), between areas of high and low need (2) and for the targeting of the most severely ill (3); as was the need for bridging money or ring-fencing of money as services move from a hospital to a community focus (2).

* The numbers in brackets indicate the number of separate reports in which the sub-themes figure (maximum = 10).

Source: Lelliot *et al.* (1997).

Jargon box

Care Programme Approach an administrative arrangement introduced in
1990 that includes (i) the allocation of a key worker, (ii) an assessment of
needs, (iii) a care plan, (iv) a care plan review meeting
section 117 of the Mental Health Act 1983 health and social services have a
duty to provide aftercare for detained service users
care management social services' equivalent of CPA: they have a duty under
the NHS and Community Care Act 1990 to provide assessment of needs
and social care
key worker professional with main responsibility for assessing needs and
delivering care
supervision register a list of the service users of each provider who are at
particular risk of harm to others, self-harm or self-neglect.

References and further reading

Audit Commission (1986) *Making a Reality of Community Care.* London: HMSO.
Challis, D. (1986) *Case Management in Community Care.* Aldershot: Gower.
Department of Health (1990) *The Care Programme Approach for People with a
Mental Illness Referred to as the Specialist Psychiatric Services,* 1990,
HC(90)23/LASSL(90)11. London.
Department of Health (1993) *The Health of the Nation.* London: Department of
Health.
Department of Health (1994) *The Health of the Nation, Key Area Handbook,
Mental Illness.* London: Department of Health.
Department of Health (1995) *Building Bridges: A Guide to Arrangements for Inter-
agency Working for the Care and Protection of Severely Mentally Ill People.*
London: HMSO.
Griffiths, R. (1988) *Community Care: An Agenda for Action.* London: HMSO.
Holloway, F. (1994) Supervision registers. Recent government policy and legisla-
tion, *Psychiatric Bulletin,* 18: 593–6.
House of Commons Health Select Committee (1994) *Better off in the Community?
The Care of People who are Seriously Mentally Ill.* London: HMSO.
House of Commons Social Services Committee (1985) Second report, session
1984–5, *Community Care,* paragraph 181. London: HMSO.
Kingdon, D. (1994) Care programme approach. Recent government policy and
legislation, *Psychiatric Bulletin,* 18: 68–70.
Lelliot, P., Audini, B., Johnson, S. and Guite, H. (1997) London in the context of
mental health policy, in S. Johnson, R. Ramsay, G. Thornicroft, L. Brooks, P.
Lelliot, E. Peck, H. Smith, D. Chisholm, B. Audini, M. Knapp and D. Goldberg
(eds) *London's Mental Health:* London: King's Fund.
Mental Health Act 1983. London: HMSO.
Mental Health (Patients in the Community) Act 1995. London: HMSO.
The National Health Service and Community Care Act 1990. London: HMSO.
NHS Executive (1994a) *Guidance on the Discharge of Mentally Disordered People
and their Continuing Care in the Community.* Health Service Guidelines.
HSG(94)27. London: HMSO.

NHS Executive (1994b) *Introduction of Supervision Registers for Mentally Ill People from 1 April 1994*, HSG(94)5. London: HMSO.

NHS Executive (1996a) *Spectrum of Care. Local Services for People with Mental Health Problems.* London: HMSO.

NHS Executive (1996b) *Guidance on Supervised Discharge (Aftercare under Supervision) and Related Provisions*, HSG(96)11. London: HMSO.

NHS Executive (1996c) *24 Hour Nursed Care for People with Severe and Enduring Mental Illness.* Leeds: NHS Executive.

NHS Executive (1996d) *Review of Purchasing of Mental Health Services by Health Authorities in England.* Leeds: NHS Executive.

NHS Executive (1996e) *An Audit Pack for Monitoring the Care Programme Approach. Monitoring Tool*, (96): 16, HSG(96)/LASSL. Leeds: NHS Executive.

Onyett, S. (1992) *Case Management in Mental Health.* London: Chapman and Hall.

Patmore, C. and Weaver, T. (1991) *Community Mental Health Teams. Lessons for Planners and Managers.* London: Good Practices in Mental Health.

Peay, J. (1998) *Criminal Justice and the Mentally Disordered.* London: Ashgate.

Peck, E., Smith, H., Barker, I. and Henderson, G. (1997) The obstacles to and the opportunity for the development of mental health services in London: the perceptions of managers, in S. Johnson, R. Ramsay, G. Thornicroft, L. Brooks, P. Lelliot, E. Peck, H. Smith, D. Chisholm, B. Audini, M. Knapp and D. Goldberg (eds) *London's Mental Health*: London: King's Fund.

Ritchie, J., Dick, D. and Lingham, R. (1994) *The Report of the Inquiry into the Care and Treatment of Christopher Clunis.* London: HMSO.

Shepherd, D. (1996) *Learning the Lessons*, 2nd edn. London: Zito Trust.

Social Services Committee The National Health Service and Community Care Act 1990. London: HMSO.

Wing, J., Beevor, A., Curtis, R., Park, S., Haddon, S. and Burns, A. (1998) Health of the Nation outcome scales (HoNOS), *British Journal of Psychiatry*, 172: 11–18.

Section B
Six key steps for developing manageable mental health services

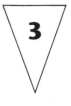

3 Step 1 The vision: agreeing the guiding principles

Key themes

In this chapter we aim to help you:

- establish a process early to identify what the service wants to achieve
- involve a wide range of local stakeholders
- recognize that differences of view are valuable
- seek consensus on guiding principles
- understand that time spent at an early stage will more than pay for itself later.

There are advantages in recognising a just principle even when events are not ripe enough for its application, when it looks Utopian and excites the derision of practical men; for it slowly modifies feelings and ideas, acts as a solvent of prejudices, and, notwithstanding seemingly insuperable difficulties, tends by hardly perceptible degrees to its realisation in action.

(Henry Maudsley, *Responsibility in Mental Disease* 1898)

Introduction

Before considering the building blocks of the separate service components, we believe it is important to ask the following questions. What is the mental health service for? What type of service do we want to offer? What is the service currently available locally? How will we know in future if the service is developing in a positive way? In other words, we suggest that you address very early on the fundamental question of which principles should

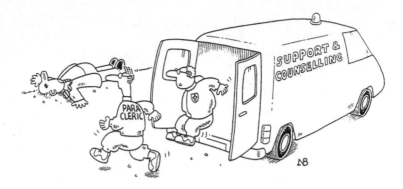

guide your service. In this chapter we shall therefore discuss the guiding principles in terms of their relation to the development of community care policies as a whole, and their direct relevance to guiding local inter-agency mental health service developments.

Establishing guiding principles for community care

A degree of consensus has been established between clinicians, planners and service user organizations in their understanding of the essential principles that should underpin community-orientated mental health services. The following summary (based on MIND Publications 1983) of principles guiding the national community care policy suggests that services should be:

- local and accessible
- comprehensive
- flexible
- consumer-orientated
- aiming to empower service users
- racially and culturally appropriate
- focused on strengths
- based on normal community supports and networks
- orientated towards meeting special needs
- accountable.

It is useful to expand upon each of these proposed principles to see what they mean:

- Services should be *local and accessible* and to the greatest extent possible delivered in the individual's usual environment. This reflects the view that most people want to continue to live in their own homes if at all possible, and that services should be organized to achieve this aim. Therefore it will usually be important that services are located within easy reach of the area they serve.

- Services should be *comprehensive* and address the diversity of needs of the individual. This principle promotes the view that the services an individual receives should try to meet the whole range of problems of that person. This will usually include a range of generic and specialist services, implying that the interfaces between the service components work for the benefit of service users.
- Services should be *flexible* by being available whenever and for whatever duration. There should be a range of complementary models that provide individuals with choice and which vary according to need.
- Services should be *consumer-orientated*, based on the needs of the user rather than those of providers, and they should be developed in consultation with the people who use the services.
- Services should *empower service users* by using and adapting treatment techniques that enable users to enhance their self-help skills and retain the fullest possible control over their own lives.
- Services should be *racially and culturally appropriate* and include use of culturally appropriate needs assessment tools, representation on planning groups, training for staff, use of indigenous workers and bilingual staff, and identification and provision of alternative basic facilities.
- Services should *focus on strengths*. They should be built on the skills and strengths of service users and help them maintain a sense of identity, dignity and self-esteem.
- Services should be *based on normal community supports and networks* by being in the least restrictive and most natural setting possible. The ordinary work, education, leisure and support facilities in the community should be used in addition to specialized developments. Therefore we suggest that specialized services should only receive investment if mainstream services are insufficient.
- Services should *meet special needs*, with particular attention being paid, for example, to those with physical disabilities, learning disabilities, the homeless or those in contact with the criminal justice system.
- Services should be *accountable* to users and carers; there should be local mechanisms at the level of individual users (such as direct involvement in care plans and complaints procedures), and for their representative groups (such as user satisfaction and preference surveys, and consultation forums), and for their advocates (such as regular provider–Community Health Council meetings).

No particular list of 'apple-pie' principles will suit every locality and so we would like to offer 'the three ACEs' scheme, which is a shorthand way to keep some of the important options in mind, as shown in Table 3.1.

To some degree the values contained in the three ACEs reinforce those described in the list earlier. The first column of ACEs begins with *accessibility*, which is a key issue from many surveys of user and carer views on deficiencies of current services. Very often they report that services are slow

Table 3.1   'The three ACEs': principles to guide community care

Accessibility	Autonomy	Accountability
Comprehensiveness	Coordination	Continuity
Efficiency	Equity	Effectiveness

Source: Thornicroft and Tansella (1999).

to respond in crisis, and offer access only to remote types of service. Many examples of this are given in the MIND survey of users' views and the King's Fund study on London's mental health services (Rogers *et al.* 1993; Johnson *et al.* 1997). Too often services fail to offer anything more than a very limited range of choice of, for example, day care services, and cannot be described as anything approaching comprehensive. Nor are they based on any data that describes how efficiently (based upon the best available evidence) they are using the resources available.

The second column of ACEs includes *autonomy*, which refers to how far the net effect of the services is to enhance independence in short and the long term, while *coordination* describes whether the various disciplines and agencies involved know enough of each other's activities to complement each other, both strategically and operationally. *Equity* means the extent to which resources are distributed in relation to need and in accordance with a locally accepted allocation that is accepted as fair.

The third set of ACEs begins with *accountability*: the quality of a service that establishes a line of reporting and responsibility to higher levels of the organization, and which in the health service will involve methods of justification to the payer (the taxed population via the Treasury) and to the proxy payer (the health authority) as to whether services represent value for money or not. Chapter 8 expands on this point. *Continuity* is one of those words more often used than clearly explained. We use it to mean the way services offer closely linked services at one point in time, or a process of care over a period of time that keeps in contact with the user without substantial gaps. *Effectiveness* refers to whether a particular type of treatment or service, in routine clinical practice rather than in experimental settings, produces benefits for users.

Using guiding principles for local inter-agency collaboration

The principles referred to in the previous section can be useful at the local level. We wish to emphasize two points here. First, we believe that the values relevant in each specific service will need to reflect local circumstances, and cannot simply be imported from another service without modification. Second, the process of establishing the guiding principles is as important as the content of the principles finally selected. In this context the overall principles need to be hardened up into local procedures and

Table 3.2   Principles of inter-agency working

Issue	*Example*
• a commitment to joint working at all levels	• bring health and social services into all relevant planning groups
• a focus on service users	• regular joint user preference surveys
• agreed and jointly 'owned strategy'	• chief officers involved and endorse agreed strategy
• agreed and well understood procedures for accessing the service	• integrated out-of-hours services
• inter-agency information exchange	• integrated case notes
• joint commissioning	• high support residential services
• a commitment to single and multi-agency training	• Care Programme Approach training
• regular review of inter-agency working arrangements	• active local Joint Planning Team

Source: Department of Health (1995: 9).

operational policies. The challenge here is to encourage or create types and styles of service embodying the agreed principles, and to redirect or decommission other services running counter to the agreed direction. Table 3.2 gives examples of features of inter-agency working which can promote the more abstract principles included in the three ACEs.

Deciding which principles are relevant locally

In everyday practice it may be necessary for staff to allocate specific time to discuss what principles should apply to your local service. This is especially important in services where staff feel they are too busy to spend time away to discuss values, because it is precisely in those services where detailed plans are needed about what services should be prioritized, and why. In other words, the most pressurized staff most need to try to agree clearly the purpose of their service. The most common way to achieve this is the 'away day', an invention which has in recent years become commonplace. In our experience this occasion is used to best effect if an external facilitator, who understands the local organizational setting in detail, meets key staff in advance. The whole group will need to appreciate that those involved will be staff who may reflect very widely differing views and values about what should be the core tasks of the service. These differences commonly fall along lines separating clinical from managerial staff, doctors from nurses, health from social service staff, and professionals from users, carers and voluntary organizations. In addition, to a considerable extent, each particular working group will be strongly influenced by powerful individuals of whatever background. One example of the results of such a process is shown in the following extract. It summarizes the principles agreed to guide

Table 3.3   Comparison between clinical and managerial approaches

	Clinical	*Managerial*
Level of interest	• individual service user assessments and interventions	• whole organizational assessments and system interventions
Key concerns	• welfare of service users • resources to deliver treatments	• welfare of the business • managing within resources
Timescale	• many years	• year on year
Job security	• externally defined (training grades)	• low or self-defined
Rewards	• service user improvement • good relations with clinical colleagues	• good fit with style and values of managerial colleagues • meeting business targets
Sources of burnout	• frustration with bureaucracy • lack of respect/value from staff • insufficient resources to practice to a minimum acceptable standard of care • untoward clinical event inquiry	• frustration with organization • poor fit between personal and organizational values • lack of respect • lack of support (senior managers and peers) • service failures • untoward clinical event inquiry • budget cuts • unchallenged unreal targets • lack of organizational clarity to effect change • lack of strategy – crisis management only (reactive/proactive)
Bottom line (resigning matter)	• minimum standards of care – clinical safety, least restrictive alternative, minimum effective dose	• clinical safety • uncontrolled overspend • insufficient resources • consequences of untoward event inquiry

the development of a general adult sector mental health team, which were negotiated before the team moved from a hospital base to a community mental health centre.

The sector team will establish a service which:

a   is *new*, both in principle and in practice
b   is based on an epidemiological understanding of local needs
c   is *community-based*, that is, aiming to preserve or strengthen service users' ties with family, friends, neighbourhood, and the wider community

d is *local, accessible, responsive,* and *accountable*

e *integrates* psychiatric care with general practice, social services and other government and non-government agencies

f provides a *range of flexible treatment options* in a variety of settings fostering the above aims

g is uniquely placed, through its intimate association with a centre of *academic excellence,* for highest quality evaluation, the national dissemination of effective models of care, and training.

Early discussions on values are also important because they can identify the common ground and the differences that will necessarily occur among members of a planning group. These value-based views will have profound effects, sooner or later, upon what the group can achieve. If an examination of values is not explicit early on, the value differences will surface at a later point and be manifested as disagreements about particular operational matters. If a framework of principles has already been established, then each subsequent disagreement can refer back to overall agreed statements of what the group is trying to achieve. Each detailed issue can then be reframed in terms of which particular service element best fits the agreed values.

Often individuals with different professional and organizational backgrounds – or different types of previous experience – will show recognizable patterns in the views they express as these differences. If used constructively, these differences can enrich the plans that develop. Some of these patterns are indicated in Table 3.3. In our experience, therefore, the time spent initially on establishing guiding principles more than pays for itself later on.

References and further reading

Beeforth, M. and Wood, H. (1996) Purchasing from a user perspective, in G. Thornicroft and G. Strathdee (eds) *Commissioning Mental Health Services,* 205–14. London: HMSO.

Beeforth, M., Conlon, E., Field, V., Hosher, B. and Sayce, L. (eds) (1990) *Whose Service is it Anyway? Users' Views on Co-ordinating Community Care.* London: Research and Development for Psychiatry.

Covey, S.R. (1992) *Principle Centred Leadership.* London: Simon and Schuster.

Department of Health (1995) *Building Bridges: A Guide to Arrangements for Inter-agency Working for the Care and Protection of Severely Mentally Ill People.* London: HMSO.

Johnson, S., Ramsay, R., Thornicroft, G., Brooks, L., Lelliot, P., Peck, E., Smith, H., Chisholm, D., Audini, B., Knapp, M. and Goldberg, D. (1997) *London's Mental Health.* London: King's Fund.

Kanter, K.M. (1992) *The Change Masters.* London: Routledge.

Maudsley, H. (1898) *Responsibility in Mental Disease.* New York: D. Appleton.

McIver, S. (1991) *Obtaining the Views of Users of Mental Health Services.* London: King's Fund Centre.

MIND Publications (1983) *Common Concern.* London: MIND.

National Institute of Mental Health (1987) *Towards a Model for a Comprehensive Community-Based Mental Health System.* Washington, DC: NIMH.

Peters, T. (1987) *Thriving on Chaos.* London: Macmillan.

Peters, T. and Waterman, R. (1982) *In Search of Excellence.* New York: Harper-Collins.

Rogers, A., Pilgrim, D. and Lacey, R. (1993) *Experiencing Psychiatry: Users' Views of Services.* London: Macmillan.

Thornicroft, G. and Tansella, M. (1999) *The Mental Health Matrix.* Cambridge: Cambridge University Press.

World Psychiatric Association (1990) WPA statement and viewpoints on the rights and legal safeguards of the mentally ill, *WPS Bulletin,* 1: 32–3.

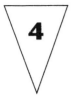

Step 2 **Estimating population needs**

Key themes

In this chapter we:

- stress the importance of planning on the basis of needs assessments
- distinguish between individual and population levels for needs assessments
- outline four methods to assess population needs
- give practical examples of how to compare actual provision with assessed need
- suggest how to establish a network of information alliances.

They also forced me to eat. They divided up the servings with the strictest sense of justice, each according to her need.

(Isabel Allende, *The House of the Spirits* 1985: 156)

Introduction

We encourage you, as a manager, to see the planning of services more as a way to move creatively towards the range of services you want to see in your area in the future, rather than as a limited exercise in minor modifications at the margins. This is a challenging way to proceed. It will require you to answer the questions: what are the levels and types of mental health problems in your area, and what are the needs of services users? In trying to answer these questions, you will need to work closely with a range of local interests, both to produce an inclusive picture of what services exist and

Table 4.1   Areas of need included in the Camberwell Assessment of Need (Phelan *et al.* 1995)

---

  1 Accommodation
    What kind of place do you live in?
  2 Food
    Do you get enough to eat?
  3 Looking after the home
    Are you able to look after your home?
  4 Self care
    Do you have problems keeping clean and tidy?
  5 Daytime activities
    How do you spend your day?
  6 Physical health
    How well do you feel physically?
  7 Psychotic symptoms
    Do you ever hear voices or have problems with your thoughts?
  8 Information on condition and treatment
    Have you been given clear information about your medication?
  9 Psychological distress
    Have you recently felt very sad or low?
 10 Safety to self
    Do you ever have thoughts of harming yourself?
 11 Safety to others
    Do you think you could be a danger to other people's safety?
 12 Alcohol
    Does drinking cause you any problems?
 13 Drugs
    Do you take any drugs that aren't prescribed?
 14 Company
    Are you happy with your social life?
 15 Intimate relationships
    Do you have a partner?
 16 Sexual expression
    How is your sex life?
 17 Child care
    Do you have any children under 18?
 18 Basic education
    Do you have difficulty in reading, writing or understanding English?
 19 Telephone
    Do you know how to use a telephone?
 20 Transport
    How do you find using the bus, tube or train?
 21 Money
    How do you find budgeting your money?
 22 Benefits
    Are you sure that you are getting all the money you are entitled to?

---

what should exist, and because the process of establishing need will be very important in influencing how far your proposed solutions will actually work in practice.

A rational approach to planning services that are fully appropriate for your local population will include the systematic assessment of the needs of the mentally ill within each catchment area. This should also include those who have severe mental health problems but are not currently in contact with services. A local case register could be used to aggregate the needs detected in all these individuals, and the services developed to fit them. However, planners in many districts do not have access to the extensive information of a case register. A more pragmatic managerial approach is to assess local needs for services by interpreting the incomplete mosaic of data that is to hand.

Needs can be measured both at the individual and at the population level. An example of an individual level needs assessment approach is the Camberwell Assessment of Need (CAN, Phelan *et al.* 1995). This is a 22-question assessment designed to identify the needs of people with severe mental illness (Table 4.1). It can be rated by a staff member, by the service user directly or by both, and has been shown to be reliable in use.

In terms of assessing needs at the population level, different types of locally available census and service-use data can be used to assess current local service needs. The methods outlined here should only be regarded as approximations that can be used as proxies for more detailed local needs assessment. However, they do provide a means of beginning to plan services in a way that is informed by the characteristics of the local population, without having to undertake further local research. The common sources of relevant information for population needs assessment are:

- ONS (Office of National Statistics, formerly Office of Population, Census and Surveys) data
- health service (performance) indicators
- purchaser strategy documents and information departments
- Audit Commission reports
- Mental Health Act Commission reports
- social services/local authority information department
- computerized sources (e.g. Mental Illness Needs Index, MINI)
- Health Advisory Service reports.

As an example of how to use such information in practice, we shall use the example of an imaginary health district, here called Planningham. Tables 4.2 and 4.3 show the main characteristics of Planningham that are referred to in the following examples.

The data in Table 4.3 illustrates an issue that is important to remember in comparing local data with national figures. There are no standard classifications for the collection of service information, and there will often be inconsistencies between data sets in the age ranges and diagnostic categories included. You need to be careful, therefore, to make sure that like is

Table 4.2   Basic information required for population-based estimation of service needs: demographic characteristics of Planningham

Census indicator	Figure for Planningham	Source of information
Population	250,000	ONS/Census
Location	inner city	maps!
Jarman index of social deprivation	39th most deprived of 400 districts	St Mary's Hospital London (Dept. of General Practice)
Ethnic mix	70% White, 15% Asian, 12% Black Caribbean, 2% Black African	ONS/Census
Homeless known to local authority	1,500 households	housing department
Street homeless	175 individuals	housing department/local surveys
Unemployment	17% economically active population unemployed	ONS/Census
Suicide rate	16.2 per 100,000 per year	health service indicators; public health staff at purchasing authority
Age structure	slight over-representation of 25- to 44-year-olds compared with national age structure	ONS/Census

compared with like. In practice accurate information on several of the categories may not be available. You then have a choice in how to proceed. You can plan ahead on the basis of any very rough estimates that are to hand, or you can commission the collection of this information and delay planning until the results are available. Another approach is to go ahead on the basis of very limited estimates, commissioning better quality data and bringing that into play at a later stage.

Simple information of the types illustrated in Tables 4.2 and 4.3 may be used to assess current local services by four main methods, each with some limitations. These four types are:

Method 1 local need may be estimated on the basis of epidemiological studies that give figures for the national prevalence of psychiatric disorders

Method 2 levels of service provision and use expected locally may be calculated from national and international patterns

Method 3 current local services may be compared with expert views on desirable levels of service provision

Method 4 the validity of estimates derived from Method 3 may be increased by using a deprivation-weighted approach. Estimates of service

Table 4.3 Mental health service provision in Planningham

Service	Planningham level of provision	Source of information
Number of people admitted at least once to hospital	1,900 people (1,400 general adult service)	provider information dept.
Admissions per annum (including readmissions)	2,820 admissions (2,110 general adult service)	provider information dept.
Number of out-patient attendances	6,500 attendances total	provider information dept.
Acute psychiatric beds	170 beds, general adult service	provider information dept.
Community psychiatric nurses for general adult service – maximum total caseload	200 service users	provider information dept.
Intensive care unit beds	3 beds	provider information dept.
Service users in regional secure unit/special hospitals	14 service users	provider information dept. and purchaser
Day centre placements – all forms of mental illness	150 places	health and social services, voluntary sector providers
Sheltered work placements	100 places	health and social services, voluntary sector providers
Places in 24-hour staffed hostels (for people aged 18–65 with mental illness)	30 residents	health and social services, voluntary sector providers
Places in day-staffed hostels	90 residents	health and social services, voluntary sector providers
Group homes	25 residents	health and social services, voluntary sector providers

need may be adjusted on the basis of current knowledge about the relationships of mental health disorders to age, sex, ethnic group, marital status, economic status and other social variables.

In this chapter, each of the above methods is explained and illustrated using the example of Planningham.

Method 1 Using epidemiological studies of the prevalence of psychiatric disorders

An estimate of local morbidity may be derived from community studies of levels of psychiatric morbidity carried out elsewhere in the UK. Table 4.5 shows the expected numbers of people with psychiatric disorders in our

Table 4.4   Main categories of mental health service likely to be required classified according to acute/emergency and long-term/continuing care (Spectrum of Care, NHS Executive 1996a)

	Acute/emergency	*Long-term/continuing care*
Home-based services	• crisis intervention for assessment and treatment • intensive home support	• case management • domiciliary support services
Day care and out-patient (ambulatory) services	• acute day hospitals • hospital casualty departments • consultation/liaison services • acute/unplanned out-patient consultations	• planned out-patient consultations • drop-in day centres • support groups • employment/ rehabilitation workshops • day centres
Residential services (a) hospital	• acute in-patient units	• long-term hospital wards • medium-secure units • high-security hospitals
(b) non-hospital	• crisis accommodation	• ordinary housing • unstaffed group homes • adult placement schemes • residential care schemes • 24-hour nursed homes

fictional district, Planningham, based on the figures for expected morbidity summarized in *The Health of the Nation*.

Survey and case identification data from inner city London suggests that about 0.7 per cent of the population at risk suffers from some form of psychotic disorder. This would suggest an expected prevalence for Planningham of some form of psychotic disorder of 1,750, compatible with the ranges in Table 4.5.

Table 4.5   Estimates of psychiatric morbidity in Planningham based on national prevalence data

	Estimated prevalence/500,000	*Estimated prevalence for Planningham (population 250,000)*
Schizophrenia	1,000–2,500	500–1,250
Affective psychosis	500–2,500	250–1,250
Depression	10,000–25,000	5,000–12,500
Anxiety	8,000–30,000	4,000–15,000

Source: Department of Health (1993).

Epidemiological data provides an overall estimate of needs in the community. It does not indicate which forms of service are needed: most people with depression or anxiety do not need referral to specialist services. However, for schizophrenia and other psychoses this data is more useful, as it may be assumed that most service users with these severe mental illnesses will need some form of long-term contact with psychiatric services.

Returning to our fictional district, Planningham's community services accommodate 200 people on community psychiatric nurses' caseloads, 150 people in day centres, and 100 people in sheltered work placements. This might cause concern when considered in relation to epidemiological data. If the estimate that there are 1,750 people with psychotic illnesses in the district is accurate, local community services do not currently have the capacity to provide for more than a small minority of these people.

Method 2 Calculating service need from national and international patterns

The work of Goldberg and Huxley (1980, 1992) may be used to compare local service use with national and international data on service utilization. Table 4.6 shows the expected Planningham levels of morbidity and of service use, based on this model's calculations of the proportion of the population using services at various levels. These figures include the elderly as well as younger adults.

Referring to the figures for Planningham, the number of people admitted at least once to a psychiatric hospital (1,500) is high compared with these estimates of service use. However, the information considered so far gives no grounds for choosing between various possible explanations, including higher than average levels of need, greater than usual willingness to admit, and shortage of services providing alternatives to admission.

Wing (1992) gives the following national figures for service users with mental disorder in contact with services per 250,000 in 1990/91. These figures include people with dementia. Again expected levels of provision for

Table 4.6   National and Planningham expected morbidity and service use

Level of service	1-year prevalence for population at risk (%)	Expected levels for Planningham (pop. 250,000)
Adults suffering from mental illness/distress	26–31.5	65,000–78,750
Consulting primary care	23	57,500
Identified by doctors as having mental illness/distress	10.2	25,500
Seen by specialist mental health services	2.4	6,000
Admitted to psychiatric hospital	0.6	1,500

Source: based on Goldberg and Huxley (1992).

Table 4.7   National figures for service use and expected Planningham figures

Type of contact	National figures for 1990/91 per 250,000 population	Expected for Planningham
Service users attending GP per annum	64,250	64,250
Service users attending out-patients per annum	2,858	2,858
Out-patient attendances per annum	8,586	8,586
In-patients on one day, stay <1 year	135	135
Acute admissions per annum	1,095	1,095
In-patients on one day, stay 1–5 years	93	93
In-patients on one day, stay >5 years	70	70
No. in local authority residential care on one day	18	18
No. in local authority long-term day place on one day	63	63

Source: Wing (1992).

the population of Planningham may be taken from this, and are shown in Table 4.7.

Planningham again has large numbers of acute admissions compared with rates predicted from national figures (2,820 admissions compared with 1,095 predicted). The number of out-patient contacts, on the other hand, is smaller than expected (6,500 attendances compared with 8,586 predicted). This pattern could be explained in various ways. One important possibility is that the out-patient service might currently be under-resourced, leading to an inability to respond swiftly to referrals. Alternatively, service users may find the out-patient service geographically inaccessible or psychologically unwelcoming, or local professionals may have limited awareness of how to make referrals to it. If such difficulties exist, the ability of the out-patient service to avert in-patient admissions may be compromised.

Wing (1992) quotes other national figures for service use on the basis of the *Local Authority Profile of Social Services for 1989/90* (Department of

Table 4.8   Use of local authority services: predicted service levels in Planningham based on national data

	LA residential	Other residential	Day centre
England	0.4/10,000 population	0.3/10,000	4/10,000
Shire counties	0.2/10,000	0.2/10,000	3/10,000
Outer London	0.5/10,000	0.9/10,000	4/10,000
Inner London	1.2/10,000	2.2/10,000	8/10,000
Planningham	30	55	200

Table 4.9   Estimated need for general adult residential provision per 250,000 population (Strathdee and Thornicroft 1992; Wing 1992)

Type of accommodation	Midpoint number of places (Wing)	Range	Midpoint number of places (Strathdee and Thornicroft)	Range
Staff awake at night				
Acute and crisis care	100	50–150	95	50–150
Intensive care unit	10	5–15	8	5–10
Regional secure unit and special hospital	4	1–10	5	1–10
Hostel wards	50	25–75		
Other staffed housing				
High-staffed hostel	75	40–110	95	40–150
Day-staffed hostel	50	25–75	75	30–120
Group homes (visited)	45	20–70	64	48–80
Respite facilities			3	0–5
No specialist staff				
Supported bed-sits	30	–		
Direct access	30	–		
Adult placement schemes			8	0–15
Total per 250,000	394	226–565	357	174–540

Health 1990). Again, these may be extrapolated to give expected figures for Planningham, assumed to be an inner city borough (Table 4.8).

Comparing these figures with the provision figures, it appears that Planningham has low levels of day centre provision compared with current national levels (150 places compared with 200 predicted from national levels). Looking at residential placements, on the other hand, suggests greater provision than is available nationally (145 places compared with 85 predicted from national levels). Service utilization data does not of course allow for a normative assessment of the services the health authority *should* have. However, managers may find it helpful to use them to get some idea whether numbers of contacts for particular components of their local services are relatively large or small compared with services elsewhere.

Method 3 What are desirable levels of service provision?

The disadvantage of comparing local services with national data is that national average service use cannot be assumed to represent ideal levels of service provision. It is also unwise to assume that the current balance between service components such as acute beds, residential services outside hospital, day care services and community services is the best possible.

The development of ways of determining optimal levels of service provision is still in its infancy, but a number of writers have contributed to the debate.

Strathdee and Thornicroft (1992) have set out targets for service provision based on a Delphi method of summarizing expert opinion in Britain, and on likely prevalences of mental illness nationally. These targets assume that services should as far as possible be community based, with community residential places and day care taking the place of institutional care. Naturally, none of these suggested levels of provision should be taken in isolation – if one component of the mental health services is underdeveloped, this is likely to lead to a higher demand on the other elements in the system (Audit Commission 1994). Wing (1992) has made similar estimates of targets for general adult residential services. These two sets of estimates are shown in Table 4.9.

Method 4 The deprivation-weighted approach to needs assessment

The above calculations of expected levels of morbidity and of service utilization in Planningham have not taken into account its particular population characteristics. This is unsatisfactory, as there is strong evidence that social and demographic factors are closely associated with rates of psychiatric disorder.

The association between psychiatric disorders and social class (particularly for schizophrenia and depression) is one of the most consistent findings in psychiatric epidemiology. The Jarman combined index of social deprivation has been shown to be highly correlated with psychiatric admission rates for health districts in the South East Thames Region (Jarman 1983, 1984; Hirsch 1988; Thornicroft 1991; Jarman and Hirsch 1992).

It thus seems reasonable to use Jarman scores to make deprivation-weighted assessments of likely local needs for services. Weightings based

Table 4.10 Deprivation-weighted estimates of required day and residential services in Planningham

Form of provision	Estimated requirement for Planningham, based on Jarman score
Total in contact with specialist services	1,602
NHS specialist residential care with night staff	230
Other residential	322
Specialist day care (four or more half days per week)	512*
Other active contact with specialist team (excluding those in above categories)	700

* including people in non-NHS residential care, of whom half are assumed also to require day care. Based on Wing (1992).

on Jarman scores may be used to estimate where each district should fall within the national ranges for desirable levels of service provision shown in Table 4.10. Nevertheless, this approach has its limitations. In any specific area, local demographic factors must also be considered in tailoring the overall approach to local conditions, including local rates of unemployment, homelessness, and the age and ethnic composition of the local population.

Fit between current services and deprivation-weighted estimates of requirements

From using this approach the gap between actual provision and estimated need for services can be calculated. Table 4.11 gives an example.

Thus this simple exercise allows us to begin to evaluate the overall pattern of service provision in Planningham. There seems to be a relatively high level of in-patient service provision, but levels of day service and community residential services are lower than estimates of what is required.

Table 4.11   Actual services, estimated needs and service gaps in Planningham

Service	Actual level of service	Estimated number required	Gap between actual and required
Acute psychiatric beds	170 beds	140 beds	+30 beds (21% above expected requirement)
Day centre or sheltered work placements – all types of mental illness	250 places	512 places	262 places (49% of expected requirement)
Places in 24-hour staffed residences (for people aged 18–65 with mental illness)	30 residents	139 residents	−130 residents (22% of expected requirement)
Places in day staffed hostels	90 residents	111 residents	−21 residents (81% of expected requirement)
Group homes	25 residents	77 residents	−52 residents (32% of expected requirement)
Local intensive care	3 beds	10 beds	−7 beds (30% of expected requirement)
Service users in regional secure unit or special hospitals	14 service users	9 service users	+5 service users (56% above expected requirement)

Table 4.12 Examples of identifying service gaps and possible actions

Problem	Possible actions
High rates of hospital admission	• audit of reasons for admission • check follow-up of discharged service users • audit CPN caseloads • check if readmitted service users are on CPA • audit length of stay • check use of ECRs • examine gatekeeping at point of admission
Many 'acute' beds used by new long-term service users	• undertake needs assessment of all those who have been in-patients for over six months • review referral routes into high-support accommodation • assess waiting times for community care assessment
Higher than expected number of residential care places and low provision of day care	• discuss with current residential care providers extending their service to include day care • audit of actual use of residential care places
Lower than expected number of people in contact with service	• review waiting times for first assessments • consider pilot joint case registers with primary care practices • consult referrers and other agencies on appropriateness and accessibility of current out-patient services • ask referrers about ease of referral to community and day care services

Again it must be noted that it is crucial to look at all the elements in local services together. If the acute bed provision were considered in isolation, it might be judged to be unnecessarily high. However, if considered in relation to the low levels of community provision, it becomes apparent that reliance on in-patient beds and high admission rates may well be a consequence of underdeveloped community facilities. It thus seems unlikely that numbers of acute beds could reasonably be reduced without considerable further development of community services.

As a manager you may then find it useful to focus in on the gaps identified by this process. You can then highlight the ways you need to address both information and service gaps that have emerged, and examples are shown in Table 4.12.

Information alliances

The central theme of this chapter is that it is feasible to use currently available information for each local area as the basis for a rational approach to planning mental health services. Our experience is that managers often do not use such an approach and instead find themselves planning and managing services basically in the dark.

There is evidence that current mental health services throughout England and Wales are often not distributed in relation to need, however estimated (Audit Commission 1994). It is thus important to develop and apply simple pragmatic approaches to assessment of local population needs. However, more fine-tuned planning of services in each local area will require investment in an information infrastructure that can monitor service performance and continue to provide relevant information to underpin future planning cycles.

Finally, it is likely that you will need the help of allies to bring together the information you need for planning purposes. These allies will enable you to have access to the breadth of information available locally. You will also start to build a network of supporters when you begin service changes. The information allies needed for planning purposes are:

- public health and planning staff at the health authority
- Trust information and planning departments
- social services planning department
- local academic departments
- the Community Health Council.

References and further reading

Allende, I. (1985) *House of the Spirits*. New York: Knopf.

Audit Commission (1994) *Finding a Place: A Review of Mental Health Services for Adults*. London: HMSO.

Department of Health (1990) *Local Authority Profile of Social Services for 1989/90*. London: HMSO.

Department of Health (1993) *The Health of the Nation*. London: HMSO.

Glover, G. (1991) The official data available on mental health, in R. Jenkins and S. Griffiths (eds) *Indicators for Mental Health in the Population*. London: HMSO.

Glover, G. (1996) Mental illness needs index (MINI), in G. Thornicroft and G. Strathdee (eds) *Commissioning Mental Health Services*. London: HMSO.

Goldberg, D. and Huxley, P. (1980) *Mental Illness in the Community*. London: Tavistock.

Goldberg, D. and Huxley, P. (1992) *Common Mental Disorders. A Bio-Social Model*. London: Routledge.

Hirsch, S. (1988) *Psychiatric Beds and Resources: Factors Influencing Bed Use and Service Planning*. London: Royal College of Psychiatrists, Gaskell Press.

House of Commons Social Services Committee (1985) Second report, session 1984–85, *Community Care*. London: HMSO.

Jarman, B. (1983) Identification of underprivileged areas, *British Medical Journal*, 286: 1705–9.

Jarman, B. (1984) Underprivileged areas: validation and distribution of scores, *British Medical Journal*, 289: 1587–92.

Jarman, B. and Hirsch, S. (1992) Statistical models to predict district psychiatric morbidity, in G. Thornicroft, C. Brewin and J.K. Wing (eds) *Measuring Mental Health Needs*. London: Royal College of Psychiatrists, Gaskell Press.

NHS Executive (1996a) *Spectrum of Care. Local Services for People with Mental Health Problems*. London: HMSO.

OPCS (1996) *National Psychiatric Morbidity Survey*. London: HMSO.

Phelan, M., Slade, M., Thornicroft, G., Dunn, D., Holloway, F., Wykes, T., Strathdee, G., Loftus, L., McCrone, P. and Hayward, P. (1995) The Camberwell Assessment of Need (CAN): the validity and reliability of an instrument to assess the needs of people with severe mental illness, *British Journal of Psychiatry*, 167: 589–95.

Strathdee, G. and Thornicroft, G. (1992) Community sectors for needs-led mental health services, in G. Thornicroft, C. Brewin and J.K. Wing (eds) *Measuring Mental Health Needs*. London: Royal College of Psychiatrists, Gaskell Press.

Thornicroft, G. (1991) Social deprivation and rates of treated mental disorder: developing statistical models to predict psychiatric service utilisation, *British Journal of Psychiatry*, 158: 475–84.

Wing, J. (ed.) (1989) *Health Services Planning and Research. Contributions from Psychiatric Case Registers*. London: Gaskell.

Wing, J. (1992) *Epidemiologically Based Needs Assessment: Mental Illness*. London: NHS ME.

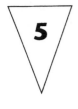

5 Step 3 Making an organizational diagnosis

Key themes

In this chapter we aim to help you:

- use a six-stage model to conduct an analysis of your organization
- identify key relationships inside and outside the organization
- spot organizational strengths and weaknesses
- identify barriers to change.

If leadership is concerned with making change happen, then the way in which you approach it will be a governing factor in whether or not you are successful.
(John Van Maurik, *Discovering the Leader in You* 1994)

Introduction

After spending time considering the policy context within which mental health services are delivered, and then taking the opportunity to map local need, it is important to make an organizational diagnosis. By this we mean a process that is a systematic appraisal of your organization. This will include assessing its recent history, the management structure, the lines of accountability, the real-life ways that decisions are made, the actual distribution of power, the organizational values, the most pressing current challenges and its overall fitness to operate.

Another way of looking at an organizational diagnosis is to see it as a map. If you are planning a journey you have never taken before you would first use a map, which shows you where you are and how to get to your destination. In organizational terms the first stage of using such an approach is to know where you are and, second, to agree on the direction of travel.

Management and senior clinical posts in the NHS are becoming increasingly complex, hence it is vital to prioritize and focus our time, energy and plans effectively. Even if you are not managing people or budgets, nevertheless you will be expected to function in a 'managed way'. A diagnosis of your organization can facilitate the development of a better understanding of your own role. You will also begin to fathom and anticipate others' expectations of you. It will help you to understand the organizational context you are working in, along with developing your ability to spot key relationships inside and outside the organization itself. Importantly, reflecting on your organization will enable you to identify organizational strengths and weaknesses and gaps in its effectiveness. We also suggest that such organizational diagnosis is not only necessary just before an individual 'rolls up their sleeves' to start a new post, it also applies before you begin a new project.

Ingredients of success and failure

We know many people (including ourselves!) who have tried to develop change programmes that were carefully thought through, and which were well managed but which somehow still failed. On reflection we think that there are often clear ingredients of success and failure. The key ingredients (according to Grant 1995) of successful projects are:

- clear goals
- understanding of the external environment
- appreciation of internal strengths and weaknesses
- effective implementation.

The factors associated with project failure are:

- over-ambitious plans or timescales
- lack of wider organizational support for the project
- the organization accepts the change but does not have the infrastructure to deliver it
- the organization accepts and delivers the change, but fails to sustain the changes
- over-dependence on charismatic leader
- limited inter-agency endorsement for the project
- lack of longer-term revenue planning.

The impact of poorly prepared change, or of unsustainable change, is devastating for any organization or business setting. It becomes even more costly when it occurs in the health care environment. As Valerie Iles has written:

One of the reasons that inappropriate changes are implemented is that the people introducing them do not adequately understand the organization they are managing. More strife has perhaps arisen at the imposition of unidimensional solutions to complex, ill defined, multifaceted, incompletely understood problems than from any other cause.

(Iles 1997: 45)

Six stages to undertake an organizational diagnosis

So how do you begin an organizational diagnosis? We suggest a simple six-stage model:

Stage 1   Before you start the job
Stage 2   The induction period
Stage 3   Gathering information
Stage 4   Checking back
Stage 5   SWOT analysis
Stage 6   Planning based upon what you have learned.

Stage 1   Before you start the job

If you are starting a new job an excellent time to begin to diagnose how the organization functions is to start before you get too immersed in your day-to-day activities. Therefore consider allocating time for this before you start the job/join the organization. Arrange if possible to go and meet your new line manager once or twice before you start the new post. This will orientate you to your new workplace and organization and to your new organization's expectations of you. It may also give you an entry into useful information on the organization, and the expectations being saved up for you when you start. We suggest that an early priority is to befriend your boss's secretary! They are often the people who really know what is going on, and will give you useful advice on how to make the best of your time with the organization, and what information may prove useful for you. There are many documents that can be gathered together for you as background reading prior to starting your job. These include:

- mission statements
- organizational strategy documents
- recent service reviews and business plans
- recent organization audit reports
- Mental Health Act Commissioner reports
- organization newsletters/staff bulletins
- minutes of meetings
- organizational structures and charts
- board minutes
- local purchaser strategy
- community care plans

- strategies from housing/social services/primary care/voluntary sector agencies
- site/service maps
- operational policies
- departmental budgets.

This information will start to show you the way the organization operates. It will also begin to highlight for you how decisions get made and who the key players are. Importantly you will begin to be able to pull out of this information the key themes and pressures currently facing the organization. This starts to give you background, context and pressure points for any task you plan to undertake when you start work with the organization.

Stage 2 The induction period

In our view a proper induction period is vital to make a fully informed start to a post, to begin building relationships (which will need to be strong to endure later tensions) and to understand your own role within the wider organization. This 'window of opportunity' is unlikely ever to return after the first few days and weeks of starting a new post. Most of the people you come into contact with will be initially intrigued by you and by your plans. We suggest that at the beginning you go into 'listening mode'. If prompted most people will start to tell you some of the organization's history, what it has done well and what has failed. They may also tell you who makes decisions, and where and how decisions get made. They may also hint at levels of morale and give clues about current concerns. People you visit initially may also describe their own expectations of your role and their view of how realistic the expectations are of the wider organization.

We recommend that you travel widely to meet your key contacts in their own offices or workplaces. Devise a list of key questions that you want answers to, but do not concentrate necessarily on getting through the whole list of questions, but rather focus on what people are saying to you. Listen for the explicit and the hidden meanings. Start with your own line manager and ask: 'What are your key priorities for me in the first six months?', 'Who are the important people for me to meet in the first few days, weeks, months?', and 'Are there any key people outside the organization I should be making links with?' On the basis of the answers to these questions, start to plan a timetable for the first part of the induction period. The key questions of organizational induction are:

- How are decisions made?
- Who has influence?
- What does the organization struggle with?
- Who controls the main budgets?
- What are the strongest pressures on the service?
- Who might I want to be wary of?

Stage 3 *Gathering information*

We suggest that as you go out and about in your work that you actively gather information. Write down what people tell you in your notebook and take away copies of any material they refer to or think would be useful reading for you. At this stage do not make any assumptions or judgements; instead, concentrate on gathering the data and setting the scene.

Ask questions of everybody and at all levels in the organization. Do not just concentrate on the obvious people like chief executives, senior managers or senior clinicians and academics. Use your time well and try to meet lots of people. When you meet them just listen and do very little talking yourself. Do not feel the temptation to tell your story or why you are there, unless they prompt you. Instead encourage them to tell you their story, to describe the organization from their perspective. Particularly try and search out those who are reluctant to speak or who would not normally have had permission to speak before, i.e. the secretaries and junior staff. We suggest that at your initial meetings you ask each of your contacts: 'Who else is it important for me to meet at the start of my job?'

Stage 4 *Checking back*

When you have spent time listening to lots of people, start to check back on the information gathered so far. At this stage we suggest that you check and cross-reference what you have been told. We expect that themes will start to emerge: are there common issues across the organization, are some parts facing issues more intensely than others, which are the central areas of achievement?

Go to colleagues (especially peers) and tactfully offer your tentative understandings. This can be useful for three reasons: you can find out whether they confirm your initial impressions, it gives an early signal to colleagues about your future views and priorities and it helps to flush out possible future allies.

Stage 5 *SWOT analysis*

After checking your first impressions you will now be prepared to analyse and assess the organization's advantages and limitations more formally. A common and often useful framework is SWOT (Strengths, Weaknesses, Opportunities and Threats). This can be made at an organizational level, but you are more likely to find this model relevant for specific projects. An example of this in practice is shown in Table 5.1.

Stage 6 *Planning based upon what you have learned*

After completing the previous stages, we suggest that you use the resulting organizational diagnosis for a number of purposes. First, use it to negotiate with your line manager or appraiser your own work targets for your first

Table 5.1   Example of a SWOT analysis – planning a new out-of-hours service

Strengths	Weaknesses
• good existing links between health and social service crisis staff • priority area for chief exec. of health authority	• no one wants to work extended hours • short-term funding only

Opportunities	Threats
• local service user group may want to link their helpline to statutory services • District General Hospital want to discuss mental health link in Accident and Emergency Department	• new GP out-of-hours service starting • overspend of neighbouring Trust may lead to a freeze of all new projects

year in post, which may necessitate the revision of your job description and key targets. Second, you can now list the projects in which you will be involved, and map out your role in each. Third, you can use this background information as you set up working groups for your areas of responsibility, in terms of personal skills of each member, their levels of political and organizational influence, and to plan contingencies for areas of weakness that you have already identified. Fourth, your analysis will help you to prioritize the use of your own time, and the time of members of your department, in terms of which activities are obligatory and which are discretionary. Fifth, your analysis can be used to 'influence up', for example to impact upon your own organization's priorities, the drafting of the local community care plan, and negotiations with purchasers. This last step may become especially important if budgetary changes during the next year mean that, owing to retrenchment you can only carry out the core obligatory tasks, which you will by now have clearly identified.

The points referred to above are more than adequate to provide an initial assessment of your organization. You may wish to review your progress in the future against your initial targets in more detail. A way of doing this is to use the information described in *Shaping Strategic Change* by Pettigrew *et al.* (1992), which is a useful reference book as all their examples are of major change projects within the NHS. In this book the authors outline the key areas in which an organization needs to be effective if it is to be ready for and receptive to change. The key areas they refer to are outlined below. We encourage managers who are interested in further organizational analysis to read the book by Pettigrew and colleagues (1992) for more details of their model and its relevance. The contexts for organizational change are:

1 quality and coherence of policy
2 key people leading change
3 environmental pressure
4 supportive organizational culture
5 managerial–clinical relations

6 cooperative inter-organizational networks
7 change agenda and its locale
8 simplicity and clarity of goals and priorities.

References and further reading

Grant, R.M. (1995) *Contemporary Strategy Analysis*. Oxford: Blackwell.
Iles, V. (1997) *Really Managing Health Care*. Buckingham: Open University Press.
Pettigrew, A., Ferlie, E. and McKee, L. (1992) *Shaping Strategic Change*. London: Sage.
Van Maurik, J. (1994) *Discovering the Leader in You*. New York: McGraw Hill.

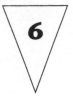

6 *Step 4* **Writing the strategic service plan**

Key themes

In this chapter we aim to show that you need to:

- involve a wide range of groups in writing the strategic plan
- allow a five-year cycle for major service changes
- plan for the whole service and then prioritize the most important early changes
- set clear tasks, and an agreed timescale and lead person for each task.

Now . . . the question may properly be asked, whether . . . we cannot recur, in some degree, to the system of home care and home treatment; whether, in fact, the same care, interest, and money which are now employed upon the inmates of our lunatic asylums, might not produce even more successful and beneficial results if made to support the efforts of parents and relations in their humble dwellings.

(Stallard 1870: 465)

Introduction

Having completed an assessment of need, and having identified your organization's strengths and weaknesses by conducting an organizational diagnosis, you now have a better informed view on what the major service gaps are, and the most pressing challenges for the service. In this chapter, rather than present abstract principles, we shall summarize a strategic plan that both of us have been involved in writing and implementing. We have added

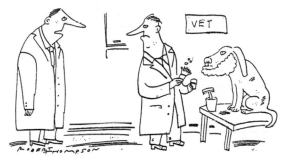

'No – I meant shave the part we're going to operate on.'

now, five years after writing the original document, a critical commentary with our own views on the strengths and weaknesses, and on what we would do differently next time.

Whatever the specific details of your own strategic plan, a wide range of agencies will need to be involved in its development, both because they have a legitimate need for involvement as providers or users of the service, or because they can block its implementation later if they are not content. If you are a manager of a mental health service provider unit, then Table 6.1 shows some of the groups you will need to consider working with, and how they may be able to contribute.

Table 6.1   Who should be involved in writing the strategic business plan?

Group	Strategy group	Involved in consultation on draft strategy	Involved in endorsement of final strategy
Provider manager	r	r	
Provider clinicians (each discipline)	r	r	r
Secretary/administrator	r		
Users and their representatives	r	r	r
Provider board members		r	r
Purchaser contracts manager	d/s		
Purchaser board members			r
Social services department locality manager/principal care manager		r	r
Director of social services		r	r
Voluntary agencies/CHC	d	r	d
GPs	r	r	r
Provider support services	s	r	d
Housing department	d	r	d
Councillors/MPs		s	s
External advisors	s	s	

Key: r = required, d = desirable, s = invited for specific issues

It is likely that in the process of establishing or extending a strategy group you will need the group to set explicit goals, with clearly identified lead people, and with a completion or reporting date for each task. We anticipate that the main task of the group will be to write a strategic service plan. To illustrate this process we consider next the business plan that has guided our work in an area of South London over the last five years. We have provided this example both to show one structure for such a plan, and to offer our own comments now on what we would do differently next time.

Case example: Camberwell sector development plan

A1 Mission

The Camberwell Sector Mental Health Service exists to help local people with severe mental health problems. It aims to develop an excellent quality service in the context of the clinical, training and research priorities of the Trust. The principles we have agreed to guide our service are set out for the next two years.

Comment

- We did not define 'severe mental health problems' at the time, and would now include in this group, first of all, service users with psychotic disorders. We would also now aim for a 'good enough' service, not for excellence, yet!
- We did not start baseline measures of quality to monitor progress towards this target.
- We did not formalize any training plan and link this clearly with the Trust Training Department's strategy.

A2 Aims for the next two years

- Establish a clear managerial and budgetary structure for the sector.
- Establish a 22-bed in-patient unit on-site in a refurbished modern ward on the hospital site.
- Acquire, refurbish and commission off-site premises for the community team base (including provision for off-site out-patient clinics).
- Use off-site premises in the community for the provision of day care combined with a drop-in centre.
- Use off-site premises for supported accommodation – eight places and two crisis-diversion beds.

Comment
- We did not pay close enough attention at this early stage to keeping the local social services department closely involved with these developments, with the consequence that the day care services became managed and financed by health rather than jointly commissioned.
- We did not base our estimates of required bed numbers on epidemiological as well as service use data, which led to problems later in terms of unacceptably high bed occupancy rates.

A3 Longer-term aims

- To provide a comprehensive and integrated mental health service to the residents of the local sector. This will include working in collaboration with social services, housing, GPs, voluntary sector, forensic, drug and alcohol and other specialist services within the Trust.
- To have established further accommodation options, with a range of community alternatives to hospital in-patient admission. These include crisis and respite facilities, for example family placement, group houses and lay community places.
- To establish with housing associations and local neighbourhood housing officers a range of 30 sheltered community residences, to include a half-way hostel, individual supported flats and group facilities, family placements and a neighbourhood helpers scheme.
- To decrease the level of crisis (unplanned emergency use of services) by 20 per cent.
- To develop a range of jointly commissioned day care, leisure, educational, social and work facilities with local social services and industry.
- To decrease the use of compulsory admissions.
- To be a national demonstration site for the implementation of the *Health of the Nation* objectives.

Comment
- These numerical goals were well meant but not useful since we did not begin any system to record this information. Also our intentions did not take into account wider changes, such as the subsequent introduction of clearer discharge arrangements, which have changed patterns of in-patient service use.
- We made the mistake of thinking that we should lead the development of supported community residential accommodation, rather than take the whole issue to the local Joint Planning Team for a inter-agency approach from the outset.

A4 The process of service development

These development plans have been agreed by all the staff teams working within the Camberwell Sector Service. We have set up working groups on accommodation, day care, nursing structure, clinical priorities, information systems, service evaluation and service models. External participation has included discussion of our plans with representatives of the health authority, Southwark Users' Forum, Joint Planning Team, the Housing Umbrella Group, social services, the Patients' Action Group, Community Health Council, local voluntary groups providing services, and the Housing Department.

Comment

- Most of these joint initiatives were achieved, but much more slowly than we had initially planned. This leads us to think that the scale of changes outlined in this chapter could reasonably be undertaken over a five-year timescale, not two years as we had thought at the outset.
- We also underestimated the slow rate of progress that is realistic when an organization and single management group both tries to implement a service change agenda and simultaneously has to continue to manage the day-to-day operational aspects of the service in transition.

B Changing the model of service

B1 Sector characteristics and current services

The Camberwell Sector Service takes referrals of adult mentally ill, under the age of 65 on first referral, who live in five specific local electoral wards. Its service provision currently centres on an acute in-patient unit of 16 beds, 120 day places for long-term service users at a day hospital on the hospital site, out-patient clinics held at the hospital, and 11 beds in a dedicated long-term in-patient rehabilitation unit.

B2 Service model and rationale

The Camberwell sector will establish a community-orientated service which:

- is *new*, both in principle and in practice
- is based on an *epidemiological* understanding of local needs
- is *community-based* – that is, aiming to preserve or strengthen service users' ties with family, friends, neighbourhood and the wider community
- is local, *accessible*, *responsive*, and accountable

- *integrates* psychiatric care with general practice, social services, and other government and non-government agencies
- provides a *range of flexible treatment options* in a variety of settings fostering the above aims
- is uniquely placed, through its intimate association with a centre of *academic excellence*, for highest quality evaluation, the national dissemination of effective models of care, and training.

A community-orientated psychiatric service, as we understand it, aims to maintain the service user's integration within his or her local community. The many functions traditionally fulfilled by a mental hospital – including treatment, occupation, social support, leisure activities, a secure home – are now to be provided in the community, as far as is possible. For service users with severe disability the principle remains, but special treatment, support and facilities are required to maximize opportunities for participation in normal life.

The model proposed is for the North and South sub-sectors each to be served by separate generic single teams, sharing a single in-patient unit. Each team would take on the full range of clinical cases appropriately dealt with at the sector level. The in-patient unit will have a dedicated ward nurse team, and all other staff members will work across settings, effectively 'following the service user' and making contact with the service user in the most appropriate setting, which may be at home, in the primary health care surgery, at day care sites or elsewhere. This model aims to offer the following advantages:

- continuity of care
- clarity for referrers to the service
- the ability to closely monitor caseload, case mix and to vary the level of contact according to clinical need
- a manageable area for the purposes of case identification, and individual needs assessment, and contact with homeless mentally ill
- very close working contact with local GPs, other primary care clinicians, housing department officers, voluntary groups, service users and their advocates and representatives.

Comment

- We notice now that we did convey to staff the principles senior staff decided should guide the service, but we did not sufficiently explain *why* these particular principles had been chosen.
- At the same time we did not assess at the start of the business planning period how far the service put these principles into practice, or assess this at any later stage. Without such an evaluation, the principles may be merely 'warm words'.

C Components of the developing service model

The following components are proposed:

- two community treatment teams
- day care facilities
- accommodation facilities
- one in-patient unit.

C1 Community treatment teams (CTTs)

The CTTs will form the core of the service model. They will provide treatment in the community as well as a range of services to the in-patient unit. There will be two special components to the CTTs' role:

1 *Assessment and treatment of acutely ill service users*: rapid response to crises, usually in the community rather than at the hospital, intensive home treatment as an alternative to hospitalization where possible, and close liaison with other community agencies. If admission is necessary, the CTT will control treatment and discharge planning throughout, and will continue to care for the service user following discharge.
2 *Rehabilitation and longer-term care of service users* with chronic and serious mental illness. The focus will be on service users with frequent admissions who have previously failed to engage with conventional out-patient services. The accent will be on assertive outreach, engagement, and home-based training in living skills.

In addition, members of the CTT will provide an out-patient service for service users with serious mental illness who are willing to attend community-based clinics, are compliant with treatment, and who do not require an intensive rehabilitation programme. Out-patient clinics will be sited in the community, either at the team base, in association with a day centre, or in primary care settings.

Comment
- Three years after the start of this business plan the crisis service was operating relatively well and community-based day care services were established, but little progress had been made to undertake home-based training in living skills for the more disabled service users.

C1.1 Team composition

One CTT is planned for each sub-sector (North, South). The boundary between the North and South teams will be based upon a survey of the places of residence of service users in contact with psychiatric services. The boundary will divide the numbers of service users between the North and South sub-sectors equally. Each team will be multidisciplinary, but with scope for the exercise of special professional expertise. A substantial part of the work will be of a 'generic' nature. A case management approach will be adopted. Each team will comprise the following types of personnel: consultant psychiatrist, specialist registrar, registrar/senior house officer, community nurses, psychologist, occupational therapist, social workers and receptionist/secretary. Some CTT services may operate across the whole sector (e.g. out-of-hours cover, psycho-educational programmes for caregivers, treatment groups for specific disorders).

Comment

- Our planning for team composition was based upon the pre-existing posts we could identify and allocate to the new sector service.
- We did not consider, in the first stage of the sector service, whether the skill mix and staff composition should be radically restructured, for example by creating community support worker posts instead of formally qualified staff positions.

C1.2 *Location*

A team base in the community is preferred, and will be sought within walking distance of the hospital. This will facilitate communication with the in-patient unit; it is also convenient to those parts of the sector with the greatest psychiatric morbidity. It is proposed that the two CTTs, although distinct, share the same team base. There are a number of advantages: some economies of scale, greater scope for support from colleagues, ready access to case records during out-of-hours cover. Adequate space might be available, but service users would need to be seen elsewhere, off the hospital site.

CTTs will also assume an important role, in conjunction with other agencies, in fostering the development of community resources for psychiatric service users. Links with voluntary agencies will be established. Integration with the in-patient unit, primary care, day care, accommodation, and other community services is central to the function of the CTTs. Support will be provided by the teams to workers employed by these agencies who deal with mentally ill service users.

C1.3 *CTT priority service user groups*

We shall use the following definitions to allocate cases to one of three categories at any one time.

High-support service user group
Individuals with severe social dysfunction (e.g. social isolation, unemployment, and/or difficulty with skills of daily living) as a consequence of severe or persistent mental illness or disorder. In particular, individuals with the following difficulties will be identified for *high levels of support*. We use the following set of categories as suggested by the Department of Health's *Health of the Nation Key Area Handbook*:

- current or recent danger to self or others
- severe behavioural difficulties
- high risk of relapse
- history of poor engagement with mental health services
- little contact with other providers of care, e.g. GP or social services
- precarious housing (e.g. bed and breakfast)
- carers who experience particular difficulty in coping with a relative suffering from mental illness.

Medium-support service user group
Individuals with a lesser degree of social dysfunction arising from mental illness or disorder, e.g. those able to work at least part-time and/or to maintain at least one enduring relationship.
   This group will also include the following individuals who are those likely to recognize, and to seek help in response to, signs of relapse, or who are those receiving appropriate services from other agencies.

Low-support service user group
Individuals who, following assessment, have been found to have specific and limited mental health-related needs that do not require extensive, multi-disciplinary input. In general, such individuals are likely to respond to brief or low-intensity intervention. This group will include, for example, service users with adjustment reaction or bereavement, or with less severe personality disorders.

Comment
- These three categories proved useful to monitor incoming referrals and to manage the caseloads of CPNs. For this purpose we allocated 3 points to each case in the high-support category, 2 points for medium support and 1 point for each low-support service user, and then added up the total number of 'points' in each CPN's caseload in discussing discharges, and who (if anyone) could take on new cases.
- We did realize early on the importance of agreeing a clear system to monitor caseload and case mix in order to manage the volume and complexity of work for community clinical staff.

C2 Day care services

We seek to provide four types of day care services: a social centre, local day care alliances, acute day care, and employment and training opportunities, and our plans are set out in Table 6.2.

Comment

This framework was useful as a way to categorize day care services, and at a later stage we conducted a user preference survey to guide the developments in terms of the location of sites, the activities to be provided and the hours of opening.

C3 Accommodation

The provision of a comprehensive community service for the severely mentally ill requires that service users have access to appropriate housing outside hospital. The present situation is that many of the service users within the community service are either inappropriately housed or are homeless. This makes readmission to hospital more likely and also increases the likely duration of admissions when they occur.

The intention of the development plan for accommodation is to prioritize the setting up of hostel accommodation for the most vulnerable service users. These will be people who are currently stranded in hospital, for want of appropriate community provision, or are at significant risk of relapse in their current accommodation. Additional places would be available for respite care, providing an alternative to hospital admission for people in the early stages of possible relapse. In the longer term it is expected that further places for service users requiring less support (e.g. flats/houses) will be developed in liaison with housing agencies.

There is an immediate need for funding of two hostels to accommodate a total of 20 people (10 in each). Each hostel will have day cover from a hostel worker. Clinical support to be provided by the sector teams. Eight beds in each hostel will be occupied in the medium term (over two years) by people who require a moderate level of support, but do not need to be in hospital. Two further beds in each will serve as respite places, for people in the early stages of relapse, for whom such an intervention is likely to reduce significantly the need for a hospital admission.

Within the current financial year we aim to acquire one of these two hostels. The success of these hostels, and the future development of less supported permanent accommodation, will depend on good working relationships with lead housing associations/agencies. Currently all accommodation development work is carried out by clinical staff, which is clearly a cost to current service levels. A housing development worker would

Table 6.2   A day care services framework

Day care type	Issue	Plan
Social centre	site preference	off-site
	number of places available	15 long-stay
	number of places required in years 1–2	15 current long-stay 15 new service users
	sector or district service	sector
	current cost	nil direct
	future cost	capital: + £80,000 revenue
Local alliances	site	current: none future: off-site, various locations, church halls, community centres, adult education centres, health centres
	management	joint, agreements/alliances development, over time but with a systematic programmed approach
	cost	capital: nil revenue: nil direct
Acute day care	site – home based – mental health centre	current: nil future: to be discussed
	management	future: direct or joint
	cost	current: nil direct future: home based – current revenue, mental health centre – to be discussed
Work services	site preference	off-site
	number of places available	20 long-stay low-skill places at hospital 10 high-skilled at day centre 3 assessment places
	number of places required for years 1–2	20 current long-stay 2 high-skilled 10 new service users 3 assessment
	sector v district service	district accessible
	current cost	hospital site: not known day centre: £70,000
	future cost	to be discussed

be able to develop the necessary community links to facilitate the above developments. This person would be likely to be seconded from an appropriate housing agency, for a minimum period of a year.

Comment

We now think that the time we spent on establishing medium-support accommodation should have been spent, from a health provider perspective, on services for new long-term service users who usually need 24-hour nurse-staffed accommodation; recent Department of Health guidance reinforces this view.

C4 In-patient services

A 22-bedded unit is required on the Trust's hospital site. The only 'ward-fixed' staff will be nursing staff (although they should be able to rotate to CTTs) and one registrar; CTT staff will continue their involvement with service users while in-patients. Consultant and senior registrar cover for the ward will be by the corresponding sub-sector doctors, while psychology, social worker and OT services will be provided by the corresponding CTT members.

Comment

One of the most difficult barriers to manage was the barrier in the imagination of staff, who did not understand the work of other teams, and so they could not effectively link with them. We therefore introduced a series of 'cross-over' opportunities for staff, including days shadowing staff in other teams, periods of several weeks or months of secondment, and a policy of rotating nursing and medical staff between in-patient and community parts of the service.

C5 Information requirements

We shall produce a list of names of service users, who have had contact with mental health services in the last two years and who live within the Camberwell sector, from the following sources:

- Hospital Patient Administration System
- the current day hospital service user register
- community psychiatric nurses' records
- admission records for the in-patient unit
- depot clinic records
- out-patient clinic notes.

Comment

The greatest problem was the relatively small number of service users' notes found by the medical records department, and the commonest reason for failure to locate records was documented as 'no notes, no tracer card'. We recommend that a temporary administrative assistant was recruited for three months to increase the number of case notes found, and to arrange their relocation to the community mental health centre.

D Linkages with local agencies and primary care

D1 *Primary care liaison*

A major objective of the Camberwell sector is to improve communication between primary and specialist care agencies. Close working relationships with local GPs, and other primary care workers, are essential in the development of an effective community mental health service. Research has consistently demonstrated that up to 20 per cent of people presenting to GPs are suffering from a mental disorder, and that GPs are the only contact for some people with serious mental illnesses, such as schizophrenia (Goldberg and Huxley 1992). This is an essential part of the sector service plan. There will be psychiatrist attachments to larger centres, with an evolving role leading to increased GP care for non-priority service user groups. We also plan to establish a nurse facilitator according to the currently favoured model of GP liaison. In the Camberwell sector links with primary care agencies are being developed by:

- weekly senior registrar clinics in local GP surgeries
- involvement of local GPs in planning meetings
- personal meetings between individual GPs and consultants to canvass views on service provision and priorities
- collection of accurate information on GP registration.

Comment

These goals were mostly achieved. Primary care arrangements have changed so quickly in recent years that you will need to give much greater attention to the views of primary care groups and ensure that they are involved in the development of the local mental health strategy.

D2 *Linkages with social services and voluntary groups*

As a service we are committed to forging and maintaining close working links with a wide range of statutory and voluntary agencies. In particular, in a local context, this means in practice Southwark Social Services and current independent providers. We shall maintain our close involvement in the development of assessment and care management procedures through the involvement of sector representatives on the Southwark Community Care Implementation Group, Maudsley Hospital Community Care Implementation Group and the Mental Health Joint Community Care Planning Group. We shall bid for mental illness-specific grant funds and Housing Corporation funds during this financial year. We shall also be closely involved with the development of specialist mental health assessment procedures within the Hospital, jointly with Southwark Social Services during years 1–2. We are now establishing working contact with local black and ethnic minority groups, user representative groups and carer representative groups.

Comment

Work with the carers of people with severe mental illness was not given a consistently high priority and remains an area needing much greater attention.

E External policy requirements and guidelines

E1 Health of the Nation targets

- To improve significantly the health and social functioning of mentally ill people.
- To reduce the overall suicide rate by at least 15 per cent by the year 2000 (from 11.1 per 100,000 population in 1990 to no more than 9.4).
- To reduce the suicide rate of severely mentally ill people by at least 33 per cent by the year 2000 (from the estimate of 15 per cent in 1990 to no more than 10 per cent).

Over the period 1985–89, local Standardized Mortality Ratios (SMRs) for suicides and undetermined deaths have been almost twice the national figure, and the age-specific rates in Camberwell are very high at all ages for men and women, except for those over 65. In terms of the actual numbers of deaths, on average each year 23 Camberwell residents die from suicide and a further 22 from injuries where the cause was undetermined. The strategy to achieve these targets will need to be developed in three areas:

- *improving information and understanding* – more extensive national and local data collection, standardized assessment procedures and clinical audit
- *developing comprehensive local services* – local joint purchasing and planning arrangements, ensuring continuity of health and social care
- *further development of good practice* – education, training, protocols and standards of good practice.

E2   Care Programme Approach

The sector service is committed to the provision of high-quality case managed continuing care where this is required by service users. We therefore plan to build upon current practice in implementing the CPA in full.

Comment

When the CPA was eventually fully introduced this did produce a significant positive change in the clinical culture, in that service users were seen in a longer-term perspective, were more likely to receive continuing offers of treatment and care, and were less likely to be overlooked and forgotten if they did not attend for services.

E3   Health authority service priorities

The local health purchasing authority has suggested the following guiding principles:

- meeting unmet need in mental health
- moving towards equity across the local boroughs
- drawing together provision across secondary care and primary care
- improving quality of care
- prioritizing users according to need
- ensuring value for money.

The most important proposed change will be better coordination between primary care, secondary care and social care, with all three components focused on community facilities. There are four different population scales on which health care services are currently provided:

- for 500,000 people upwards   regional secure unit, specialist child services
- 150,000–300,000 population   acute beds, intensive care beds, social services
- 35,000–75,000 population   sector community mental health teams
- fewer than 20,000 people   primary care.

A shift towards local community mental health teams is envisaged because community care is gradually replacing in-patient care as the main service. In-patient beds can be regarded as a back-up facility rather than the main service focus. The community level sectors imply centres that are more closely identified by both service users and general practitioners.

Comment

We realized that it was very important to have a close working relationship with the purchasing authority mental health contracts manager, both for the ongoing contractual cycle, and to be able to respond quickly to any other bidding opportunities or financial threats that arose.

E4 NHS and Community Care Act

Staff within the Camberwell sector have taken the lead within the hospital on the planning and implementation of the Assessment and Care Management aspects of the Act, and will continue with these important statutory responsibilities. In addition we shall develop our service in accordance with the good practice guidelines set out in the Southwark Community Care Plan Priorities, the Patient's Charter, and locally agreed Quality Assurance and Nursing Standards.

F Resources required

As part of its development, the Camberwell sector will require continuing and changing support from the various clinical and non-clinical support services within the Trust.

F1 Clinical services

A new relationship between sectorized and general adult services in the Community Division and the centralized Community Division Clinical Services remains to be fully and satisfactorily clarified and formalized in terms of funding, referral protocols and activity. It is expected that this clarification will be in terms of service level agreements and external contracts. Of particular concern are:

- forensic services
- psychology
- psychotherapy
- eating disorders
- mentally ill people with learning disabilities
- mother and baby services
- drug services
- alcohol services
- intensive care unit
- special care unit.

F2   Nursing directorate

A service level agreement is in progress for professional advice regarding quality standards for community nursing, together with agreed audit procedures and follow-up by suitably experienced nursing personnel. Supervision of senior nursing staff will also need to be agreed.

F3   Central clinical support services

- *Pharmacy*: service level agreements specifying cost and volume of drugs used together with levels of professional pharmacy advice and inputs from a community pharmacist. It would be expected that pharmacy advice would be available in local settings at agreed weekly times, as well as more generally over the telephone.
- *Pathology*: service level agreement similar to pharmacy specifying in particular different timescales available, with different charges for return of test results.
- *Patient services*: these will increasingly be required at a regular time at community locations. Ambulatory welfare and Mental Health Act services would prove invaluable in providing a service that does not entail visits to the hospital site.
- *Placement services* and advice on Care in the Community will also need to be subject to a service level agreement.
- *Radiology and EEG*: will continue to be provided at the main hospital site. Results will need to be transported to the Camberwell sector team base.

The sector intends increasingly to involve service users and professionals in the work of the sector teams, with specific earmarked individuals who may in due course become members of those teams.

F4   Central non-clinical support services

- *Information services*: the sector is critically dependent on detailed clinical information for the most effective delivery of care. In the short term it needs support in creating its own service user database. The sector requires to be consulted in agreeing the project's user requirements. This should include the uploading of data collected for clinical services prior to implementation.
- *Medical records*: as service users are referred from the Depot Clinic, the sector will seek additional resource to support its own teams. Once again earmarked individuals will need to be available to undertake off-site clinics. The provision of a proper medical records facility that is maintained and supported will require the reallocation of existing medical records staff and duties.
- *Transport*: the development of a comprehensive transport service between sector bases and services is critical to the success of the sector. Many items

will need to be transported, and the service development department is being commissioned to produce a tender specification as the geographic spread of services becomes apparent.

- *Catering*: provision of food is a recurrent concern. Considerable work will need to be undertaken to ensure that food is provided, and that the current kitchens can supply the food subject to proper transport arrangements being in place.
- *Cleaning*: additions to the existing contract will be needed to ensure proper cleaning services are in place.
- *Works*: tenders need to be prepared for properties being purchased and used by the sector. It is envisaged that the works department will tender for these alongside private contractors. These tenders will also encompass security.
- *Supplies*: requisition points will need to be set up in each new sector service off-site. There is a further transport issue regarding the proper delivery of supplies.
- *Site services*: these are currently provided on a hospital basis but will be needed by individual sites. Services include photocopying, key holding and ordering transport.
- *Quality and clinical audit*: will continue to provide untoward incident reporting and other services.
- *School of Continuing Education*: the increased focus of the new nursing diploma in community nursing is welcomed. Access to places needs to be clarified.
- *Management accounts*: will continue to provide budget reporting services and budgetary advice as currently, but with dedicated staff for sector purposes.
- *Financial accounts, creditor payments, payroll*: no change is envisaged in the service.
- *IT services*: PC and software support is particularly vital and will be needed at increasingly dispersed locations.
- *Estates*: Estates will provide advice on surveying and purchasing property, design, health and safety and refurbishment of existing and new properties. In addition Estates will liaise on additional architectural advice.
- *Marketing and contracting*: in particular, advice will be sought on extra contractual referrals both internally and externally, and on the presentation of sector services (for example to GP fundholders) within the corporate marketing strategy.
- *Service development*: this department will provide project management for major capital projects, prepare tender documents for subcontracted services, and advise on accessing funding for housing projects. It will provide ad hoc advice and coordination of projects that emerge during the course of the move to the community, with greatly strengthened clinical input.
- *Selection and recruitment*: medical staffing; employee relations; training

and development; occupational health; manpower services: the changes envisaged in these services as a direct result of sectorization are to link central staff more directly with the service needs at the sector level.

Comment

- We underestimated the importance of good working relations with non-clinical support services, and while some of these services adapted to community sites very flexibly, others continued to act as if they only had responsibility for those activities taking place on the main hospital site. Open days, meetings at the new sites, and some incentives for these services to gain credit and reward for supporting community services would have helped.
- It is important also to maintain close contact with senior officers within provider trusts, so that they are briefed early about developing problems, to continue to keep their trust, to try to ensure that they will be sufficiently supportive when real difficulties occur, and to access their own experience and advice.

Conclusion

In this chapter we have used the example of Camberwell to illustrate local strategic service planning, to show you how this worked in practice, and to reflect a few years later which elements worked and which did not. In our view it is very important to be as specific as possible on key definitions, for example of the service user groups to be served, and to set clear tasks and timescales, with nominated members of staff for each task. We have chosen to illustrate the process of developing a strategy at the sector level; in this case it will be vital to have the plan endorsed at Trust board level before taking the draft plan to local purchasing authorities to see if they will support it.

We think now that in addition to producing this strategic business plan we could have produced a short summary version (for example a two-page leaflet) for wider distribution within the sector service and to other local interested groups and staff. This would have included information about the planned changes and a request for comments and feedback about the plans, to win over opponents or the doubtful and to prepare the way for the implementation of the changes.

References and further reading

Goldberg, D. and Huxley, P. (1992) *Common Mental Disorders. A Bio-Social Model.* London: Routledge.

Handy, C. (1976) *Understanding Organisations.* London: Penguin Books.

NHS Executive (1996) *24 Hour Nursed Care for People with Severe and Enduring Mental Illness.* Leeds: NHS Executive.

Smith, H., Kingdon, D. and Peck, E. (1996) Writing a strategy, in G. Thornicroft and G. Strathdee (eds) *Commissioning Mental Health Services*. London: HMSO.

Stallard, J. (1870) Pauper lunatics and their treatment, *Transactions of the National Association for the Promotion of Social Science*, p. 465.

Step 5 **Delivering the service components**

Key themes
- Mental health services should provide the ten key components discussed in this chapter.
- Mental illness is so common that it is essential to set clear priority groups for specialist (secondary) mental health services.
- The boundary between primary and secondary care is therefore a crucial interface.

Introduction

Community-orientated mental health services can be defined as:

> the network of services which offer continuing treatment, accommodation, occupation and social support and which together help people with mental health problems to regain their normal social roles.
> (Strathdee and Thornicroft 1997: 513)

The development of community services has had two consistent themes: that services should be directed to *meeting individual needs* and that the traditional inherited service systems dominated by large institutions should be replaced with a more balanced and *flexible range of alternative services*. In relation to community-orientated mental health services (as defined above), this chapter focuses on the ten components of community services. The categories described are not mutually exclusive and, as in any local settings, the organization and form of services should be built on local

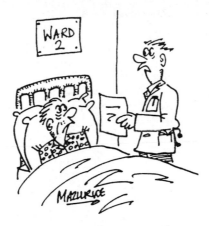

*'You've got something extremely rare,
Mr Watson – a hospital bed'*

information and circumstances, and will necessarily be more messy than this idealized list. The ten core components are:

1 case registers
2 crisis response services
3 hospital and community places
4 assertive outreach and care management services
5 day care
6 assessment and consultation services
7 carer and community education and support
8 primary care liaison
9 physical health and dental care
10 user advocacy and community alliances.

Case registers

Only a proportion of the severely mentally ill come into contact with the psychiatric services, and a sizable number of these lose contact. Research has shown that three-quarters of service users with a diagnosis of schizophrenia who were discharged from London mental hospitals had seen their GP in the year after discharge, but that less than 60 per cent had attended hospital out-patient clinics. Similarly, the South Camden schizophrenia study (1996) identified that only three-fifths of the known individuals with schizophrenia in the area were in contact with the psychiatric services. A long-term outcome of a group of depressed service users found that over half had lost contact with the hospital services; those out of contact included some of the most severely ill.

A local case register is also often useful to identify service users with the most severe disabilities related to mental illnesses. The ethical and confidentiality issues before setting up a register should be addressed at the local level. The user advocacy group MIND has identified appropriate safeguards in a 1991 policy paper. Two important further information issues are the compilation and widespread circulation of accurate and updated street lists naming the responsible team for each address, and a well indexed directory of services to allow agencies to cross-refer. The use of registers is now likely to become very much more important as services are required by the Department of Health to identify and offer continuing support and supervision to the service users at risk of harm to themselves and others.

Crisis response services

The aim of the services should be to enable the client, family members and others to cope with the emergency while maintaining to the greatest extent the client's status as a functioning community member (Phelan *et al*. 1995). The services may need to be available on a 24-hour, 7-day basis, manned by experienced mental health professionals and known to providers, families, service users, GPs and the community. Immediate psychiatric consultation should be available for rapid evaluation, diagnosis and chemotherapeutic interventions as indicated.

Indeed adequate, early treatment – associated with client, family and staff education and training – can prevent the onset of many crises. Because of the episodic nature of the illness, however, there will be instances that require acute care and rapid response crisis stabilization services. Traditionally, provision of crisis intervention has been through consultation at the local general practitioner's surgery and (in many districts) the accident and emergency departments of general hospitals. With the development of community services this has been extended by a range of options that include 24-hour telephone helplines; walk-in emergency clinics; community mental health centres; mobile outreach crisis intervention teams; community crisis residential beds for temporary respite care outside the normal residential environment when needed; and in-patient beds in a variety of settings, such as the psychiatric units of a district general hospital. The characteristics of a successful crisis service are:

• prompt access for referrers
• clear criteria for referral
• a range of treatment options (e.g. hospital, crisis house admission, intensive home treatment)
• coordinated multi-agency working (e.g. mental health service, GP, social services and casualty department)
• a commitment to inform and involve families and other carers
• an agreed triage system to prioritize service users
• set standards for response times and performance targets
• practical routine risk assessment procedures

- staff safety policies
- a clear short-term care plan
- the provision of immediate treatments that are evidence-based.

Hospital and community places

For modern-day mental health services to work, a wide range of hospital and community beds or places are necessary and interrelated. These should include secure facilities for mentally disordered offenders; well-staffed units in hospital and the community for those with challenging behaviours; acute hospital beds and a range of community beds for crisis diversion, quarter- and half-way hostel purposes; respite facilities; residential and permanent accommodation.

Acute treatment facilities should be available to provide assessment by a multi-disciplinary team; investigation facilities, to exclude an organic basis for a mental health disorder; supportive counselling and psychotherapeutic treatment; mechanisms for the provision and monitoring of medication to ensure education, maximal therapeutic effectiveness and a range of residential facilities. The location of such services has been the subject of major debate. Particular attention has been paid to the question of the role of the hospital and the appropriateness of alternative facilities including hospital hostels, home-based teams and pre-admission facilities.

The practices covered by the term 'respite care' are of increasing importance in mental health service provision. Such respite care provides relatively brief planned periods of residential care, usually of between one week and one month, during which time the service user may be fully reassessed, treatment can be modified, the family can benefit from relief from the burden of care, and the service user may be given temporary sanctuary from the demands of everyday life, which may include an emotionally charged atmosphere at home. Respite care has been most fully developed for people with learning difficulties, with physical disabilities and for the elderly. While there is evidence of substantial benefits for service users and their carers, respite services are as yet poorly developed within mental illness service provision, and await full evaluation.

The success of community-based services is crucially related to the nature and availability of accommodation with appropriate levels of support. Within the British context, a ten-tier typology of sheltered housing for people with severe psychiatric disorders has been developed by Professor John Wing (Wing and Furlong 1986):

1 unsupervised housing, where the individual lives alone or with family or friends, and contact with psychiatric services is through non-residential staff
2 as above, with a degree of administrative protection, for example from eviction for arrears in rent

3 supervised housing providing regular domiciliary supervision by a mental health practitioner
4 group homes where several residents with psychiatric disorders share the same house, perhaps supervised by a residential landlady, with support from visiting staff
5 supervised hostels where residents may each have a bedroom and share communal facilities
6 hostels with residential staff offering close daily supervision
7 as number 6, with a higher level of supervision for residents more disabled by psychiatric or physical conditions
8 hostel accommodation supplemented with night nursing staff, the provision of meals and the supervision of budgeting
9 for those with severe challenging behaviours, intensive supervision may be needed, with high staffing levels
10 a basic nursing unit for people who are incontinent, immobile or disorientated.

To ensure the success of community housing provisions, liaison with community members and caring agencies is essential. Community hostels should be within easy access of shops, sports facilities, cinemas, day centres, workshops and pubs; a clear plan for medical cover should be formulated before the admission of residents; there should be detailed discussion with all staff members (especially GPs, if they are to be involved), with agreement about spheres of responsibility, emergency work, prescribing and communication. Aside from permanent housing, homeless individuals who are mentally ill will require additional living situations with varying degrees of supervision and structure, including emergency shelters.

Mental illness rates in the homeless range from 41 to 93 per cent, alcohol dependency in over 60 per cent, and chronic medical and dental problems in over 40 per cent of this group (Scott 1993). These individuals characteristically have restricted social support networks, little contact with psychiatric services, lower readmission rates than their domiciled counterparts, and little likelihood of referral to long-term care facilities. Local psychiatric facilities clearly do not serve these homeless mentally ill at all adequately. Even so, it is important to avoid over-generalizations about the homeless mentally ill; studies show considerable variations, for example in the proportion of such people who come from the local area.

Assertive outreach and care management services

Since the early 1960s a number of studies have compared acute home-based care with hospital care. Despite differences in the models and evaluative methodologies used, these studies confirm a decrease in hospital admissions, improvement in clinical outcome and social functioning, and greater service user satisfaction from acute home-orientated care. Reviews of the community-orientated approach to continuing care have shown that outcome from assertive outreach programmes is in no published case worse than for standard hospital-based treatment, and is often better. To date, however, these studies have not indicated which sub-groups among the seriously mentally ill may be most and least likely to benefit from these forms of care. Further, the major outcome variables of these studies are often service usage indices. There are a number of different models of case management. The direct care-giver variants of case management emphasize the staff–service user relationship as the key component through which effective care is channelled, in the tradition of social case work. Brokerage models, however, give the case manager a central, distant coordinating function without any necessary direct contact with the service user.

Substantial research has now investigated the outcomes of this community care policy, and the evidence is that community-based psychiatric services are as good or better than the older hospitals on all the measures that have been used (Braun *et al.* 1981). Indeed, when service users themselves and their families are asked for their preferences, they overwhelmingly favour community to hospital care (Leff *et al.* 1990). A number of experimental services have been evaluated. A controlled study in South London (Muijen *et al.* 1992) compared comprehensive assertive home-based care with standard in-/out-patient care for service users with severe mental illness. Though social and clinical outcomes were similar, service users and relative satisfaction was higher in the group receiving home-based care, and costs were lower.

Day care

Day hospitals were begun in Britain in 1946 after their establishment in the Soviet Union a decade earlier. They can be considered as either acute or daily attendance at long-term day hospitals, where the former can provide a service that compares favourably with standard in-patient treatment for some people in acute relapse. Unless day hospitals are especially orientated to the needs of the severely mentally ill, however, they can easily drift to admit service users who staff find more pleasant to work with, so that the more disabled service users are left to resort to the usually less well-staffed social services-funded day centre. In the last 20 years many day care facilities have moved away from large institutional sites as one aspect of deinstitutionalization. In addition the working of the NHS and Community Care Act 1990 has allowed day care facilities to be included in the formulation of inter-agency agreements formalized as local community care plans. The main categories of day care and their functions are:

Day hospitals

- alternative to admission for the acutely ill
- provision of support in the transition between hospital and home
- source of long-term structure and support for those with severe disabilities

- brief intensive therapy for those with personality difficulties, severe neurotic disorders and those who require short-term focused rehabilitation
- an information, training and communication resource.

Day centres

- social centres offering drop-in facilities and befriending
- work training and job preparation
- link with mainstream work, leisure and social facilities (e.g. church halls, community centres, adult education centres, health centres)
- advocacy and welfare benefits advice
- non-specialized counselling
- practical assistance with domestic tasks.

The future development of day care is likely to feature the following issues: the emergence of acute day hospitals as genuine alternatives to admission to acute in-patient wards, or to follow immediately after discharge to reduce length of stay in wards; the development of supported and transitional employment schemes to mainstream full- or part-time jobs; the growth of the independent sector as providers of job coaching and work preparation projects; the recognition of crèche and child care for day care attenders; joint arrangements between social services and the employment and education departments, including ongoing adult education opportunities.

Assessment and consultation services

Until the past few decades the majority of consultation services were conducted in hospital out-patient settings. Two innovations in community provisions have begun to redress these deficiencies. First, there has been an evolution of out-patient clinics away from hospital sites and the establishment of consultation clinics in primary care settings. Nineteen per cent of all consultant general adult psychiatrists in England and a half of Scottish psychiatrists work in this way. The evidence indicates that these clinics enhance continuity of care, particularly when the psychiatric team work in an integrated manner with their primary care colleagues. Additional advantages are that service users prefer the accessibility and non-stigmatizing setting of their local surgery; the GPs enhance their knowledge of psychiatric disorders and treatment techniques; and the mental health team have increased access to community resources and are better placed to intervene at an earlier stage in the development of illness and relapse.

Second, a growing number of community mental health centres have been established, with over three-quarters of England now served, at least in part, by such centres. The American community mental health centres attempt to provide five services; in-patient, out-patient, partial hospitalization, emergency services, consultation and education. In the UK they function more as a resource for crisis intervention, coordinating multi-disciplinary teams and as consultation services.

Carer and community education and support

Much caring of the mentally ill is done by relatives, although not all carers are blood relatives or spouses by any means: some of the most successful caring relationships are made by friends, landladies or home helps. People with schizophrenic illnesses show a severe reduction in regular social contacts, down from a norm of perhaps 30 people to only four or five. In this situation carers share the problems and difficulties of their relatives. The process of daily care for relatives who have severe social and behavioural disturbance takes place at the cost of disruption to family routine, resulting physical and psychological morbidity to the health of the other family members, and costs to the economic viability of the family unit. A recent survey of carers of this group found that practical help was often forthcoming (e.g. housing, financial advice), but that emotional help was always deficient. The commonly occurring issues for carers of people with mental illness are:

- medication management
- underactivity of the service user or isolation of the carer
- guilt and lack of information on causes of the disorders and the outlook
- worry about what will happen when the carer dies or becomes frail
- anxiety and depression of the carer
- information on accessing local services
- what to do in a crisis
- concern about suicide risk for the mentally ill relative
- linking to self-help carers' groups.

There should be assistance to families that provides education on the nature of the illness, consultation and supportive counselling on handling daily problems and intermittent crisis situations, appropriate involvement in the treatment planning process, respite care and referrals to family support groups and advocacy organizations such as the national or local mental health associations. In addition, in order to facilitate community integration and acceptance, practical support and education should be available to landlords, employers, educationalists, community agencies and others.

Primary care liaison

In Britain a powerful primary care tier of care exists that is uncommon in many other economically developed countries. About one-quarter of adults have a mental health problem of sufficient severity to interfere with some aspect of their lives in the course of a year, but only a small minority of 2 per cent are seen by specialist services (Goldberg and Huxley 1992). Typically, of 100 adults in any local area population,

- 25 have a moderate or severe mental health problem in any year
- 23 attend their GP for some reason (including physical illness)
- 14 have mental illness identified by GPs
- 2 are referred on to specialist mental health services
- 0.6 are admitted to psychiatric hospital.

While the majority of mental health disorders fall within the less severe or 'neurotic' areas, of those individuals identified as having a mental health disorder, one-tenth have a chronic disorder defined as continually present for one year or as requiring prophylactic treatment. The mental health services must develop effective ways to liaise with primary care services.

The three mental health professions most often undertaking clinical sessions in primary care are psychologists, community psychiatric nurses and counsellors.

Clinical psychologists working in primary care are significantly more likely than CPNs or practice counsellors to be referred service users with psychosexual problems, eating disorders, phobias and obsessive compulsive disorders. Service users usually report a high degree of satisfaction with their treatment (usually behaviour therapy), which can result in decreased drug prescribing.

Where psychologists have used their specialist training in cognitive therapy to treat depression, studies have found a significantly greater improvement compared to GP treatment alone, albeit with no difference three months after completion of treatment. It has been suggested that the most important role for clinical psychologists is to provide education and consultative liaison for the GP and consultation for self-help or other voluntary sector organizations.

The attachment of community psychiatric nurses to particular general practices has followed two general models (Ford 1995). In those services where the nurses are hospital based and work as members of the secondary care team, 80 per cent of their referrals are from psychiatrists whose workload is mostly made up of individuals with severe and continuing mental health disorders. In the second model, the nurses are employed by secondary care services and are attached to a particular GP. Here the referral pattern shifts, with 80 per cent of their referrals coming direct from GPs. In the latter model the caseloads are characteristically large, composed of service users with neurotic and adjustment disorders; large numbers of service users only receive care from the CPN. Although the caseloads of both the hospital based and primary care based CPNs remain similar in terms of the numbers of individuals with schizophrenia, the mean time in contact with psychotic service users is a third of the time spent with non-psychotic service users, and is almost entirely limited to the administration of injections.

In 1992, half of the employed counsellors had specialist training in counselling, but in one-fifth of instances the employing GPs were unaware of the qualification of the counsellors in their practices. Counsellors are referred a wide variety of problems ranging from family and relationship difficulties to drug and alcohol abuse and psychiatric illness (Roth and Fonagy 1996). The introduction of properly trained counsellors into primary care has been demonstrated to reduce psychotropic drug prescribing, GP consultation rates and referrals to psychiatrists, as well as providing service users and GP satisfaction.

Physical health and dental care

Service users treated in the community are often the most severely ill and vulnerable, and have significant requirements for physical as well as psychiatric care. In a study of 145 long-term users of hospital and social services day psychiatric facilities, 41 per cent suffered medical problems potentially requiring care. Therefore it is important to liaise with the providers of medical care, most often the primary care doctors. This aspect of need is helped when services are linked to the general hospital.

User advocacy and community alliances

The importance of advocacy and user involvement at all levels within services has been increasingly acknowledged. At the individual clinical level, active participation can include having access to documentation and involvement in goal-setting and reviews. Involvement of users at all stages of the planning process may facilitate alliances between professionals and their service users and bring about more effective implementation of the services. User participation in the monitoring and management of the service and in training and education are also important areas. Users' charters emphasize the rights of service users to privacy, consultation, information and choice. Mechanisms to inform individuals and their families of their legal rights are the responsibility of the services.

Over the past ten years there has been an increasing research interest in the views of individuals using general health and hospital services. Studies in the area have revealed some interesting findings, and a detailed picture of a user perspective on health care is gradually being built up. Individuals using hospital and related services for physical disorders are, on the whole, satisfied with the care they receive. Despite this, the recent increased uptake of alternative therapies may indicate a level of dissatisfaction with more traditional services. In the area of mental health the need to consult widely with users is increasingly recognized, and relevant methodologies are being developed. However, little work has been done that specifically addresses the ascertainment of users' views on the provision of primary care mental health services. These themes are developed further in Chapter 13.

Conclusion

The widespread transformation of mental health care systems – as in the last 20 years in both the US and Europe – is no new phenomenon. Such

Table 7.2   The basic service profile

Basic component	*Variations*
1 Out-patient and community services 1a home visits 1b out-patient services 1c consultation in general hospitals	• mobile services for crisis assessment and treatment (including evening and weekend services) • out-patient services for specific disorders or for specialized treatments
2 Day services (including occupational/vocational rehabilitation)	• sheltered workshops • supervised work placements • cooperative work schemes • self-help and user groups • advocacy services • training courses • club houses/transitional employment programmes
3 Acute in-patient services	• specialized units for specific disorders (e.g. intensive care and forensic) • acute day hospitals • crisis houses
4 Longer-term residential services	• unsupervised housing with administrative protection • supervised housing (boarding out schemes) • unstaffed group homes • group homes with some residential or visiting staff • hostels with day staff • hostels with day and night staff • hostels and homes with 24-hour nursing staff
5 Interfaces with other services (e.g. health, social and non-governmental agencies)	*health services* • forensic services • old age services • learning disability/mental handicap services/mental retardation • specialized psychotherapies • general physical and dental health • primary care and general practitioners *social services/welfare benefits* • income support • domiciliary care (e.g. cleaning) • holiday/respite care *housing agencies* • unsupervised housing/apartments *other government agencies* • police • prison • probation *non-governmental agencies* • religious organizations • voluntary groups • for-profit private organizations

rapid system changes were common in the last quarter of the nineteenth century when our predecessors established the psychiatric institutions. The challenge for managers and clinicians today is, in this cycle of transformation, to measure accurately the effects of interventions and service changes in order to produce a modern network of community mental health services. In developing such a network how can you prioritize which developments should take place first? This will necessitate making a distinction between the *basic components* of the service that need to be provided first of all, and then the *variations* or *alternatives* that can be considered after the basic building blocks of the service are in place (see Table 7.2). The challenge for managers, therefore, is to deliver the key components, to improve current services, to manage the local politics of the interfaces between service components, and to set priorities for which of these many tasks should be done first.

References and further reading

Berry, D., Szmukler, G. and Thornicroft, G. (1996) *Living with Schizophrenia – the Carers' Story*. Video and accompanying booklet. London: PRiSM, Institute of Psychiatry.

Braun, P., Kochansky, G. and Shapiro, R. *et al.* (1981) Overview: deinstitutionalisation of psychiatric patients, a critical review of outcome studies, *American Journal of Psychiatry*, 138: 736–74.

Ford, R. (1995) Mental health nursing and case management, in C. Brooker and E. White (eds) *Community Psychiatric Nursing: A Research Perspective, Volume 3*. London: Chapman and Hall.

Goldberg, D. and Huxley, P. (1992) *Common Mental Disorders. A Bio-Social Model*. London: Routledge.

Harvey, C., Pantelis, C., Taylor, J., McCabe, P. *et al.* (1996) The Camden schizophrenia surveys. II. High prevalence of schizophrenia in an inner London borough and its relationship to socio-demographic factors, *British Journal of Psychiatry*, 168: 418–26.

Holloway, F. (1988) Day care and community support, in A. Lavender and F. Holloway (eds) *Community Care in Practice*. Chichester: Wiley.

Johnson, S. and Thornicroft, G. (1993) The sectorisation of psychiatric services in England and Wales, *Social Psychiatry and Psychiatric Epidemiology*, 28: 45–7.

Kendrick, A., Sibbald, B., Burns, T. and Freeling, P. (1991) Role of general practitioners in care of long term mentally ill patients, *British Medical Journal*, 302: 508–11.

Leff, J., O'Driscoll, C., Dayson, D., Wills, W. and Anderson, J. (1990) The TAPS Project 5. The structure of social network data obtained from long stay patients, *British Journal of Psychiatry*, 157: 848–52.

MIND (1991) *MIND's Policy on Case Registers*. London: MIND.

Muijen, M., Marks, I.M., Connolly J. and Audini, B. (1992) Home based care and standard hospital care for patients with severe mental illness: a randomised controlled trial, *British Journal of Psychiatry*, 304: 749–54.

Phelan, M., Strathdee, G. and Thornicroft, G. (1995) *Emergency Mental Health Services in the Community*. Cambridge: Cambridge University Press.

Rogers, A., Pilgrim, D. and Lacey, R. (1993) *Experiencing Psychiatry: Users' Views of Services*. London: Macmillan.

Roth, A. and Fonagy, P. (1996) *What Works, for Whom? A Critical Review of Psychotherapy Research*. New York: Guildford Press.

Scott, J. (1993) Homelessness and mental illness, *British Journal of Psychiatry*, 162: 314–24.

Strathdee, G. and Thornicroft, G. (1992) Community sectors for needs-led mental health services, in G. Thornicroft, C. Brewin and J.K. Wing (eds) *Measuring Mental Health Needs*. London: Royal College of Psychiatrists, Gaskell Press.

Strathdee, G. and Thornicroft, G. (1997) Community psychiatry and service evaluation, in R. Murray, P. Hill and P. McGuffin (eds) *The Essentials of Postgraduate Psychiatry*, 513–34. Cambridge: Cambridge University Press.

Thornicroft, G. and Bebbington, P. (1989) Deinstitutionalisation: from hospital closure to service development, *British Journal of Psychiatry*, 155: 739–53.

Wing, J.K. and Furlong, R. (1986) A haven for the severely disabled within the context of a comprehensive psychiatric community service, *British Journal of Psychiatry*, 149: 499–58.

8 ▽ Step 6 Review and evaluation

Key themes

In this chapter we aim to:

- explain the meaning and importance of evaluation
- convince you of the relevance of service evaluation
- define efficacy, effectiveness and efficiency
- describe the most common research methods
- demystify key jargon terms
- identify the main sources for seeking information
- give ideas on how you can conduct your own service evaluation.

Intellect has a keen eye for method and technique but is blind to aim and value.

Albert Einstein

Introduction: what is evaluation?

There is now an increasing emphasis on service evaluation, yet managers do not often evaluate what they do nor the services that they provide. The view that they are usually better at action than at reflection is a commonly held one. How can the need to evaluate be reconciled with the demand on health service managers to fulfil financial targets and contracts? It is important to appreciate that the systematic scrutiny of health services is essential for managers to decide whether they are achieving what they are meant to achieve. Evaluation has been defined as 'the critical assessment,

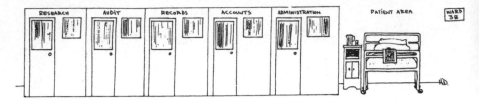

on as objective basis as possible, of the degree to which entire services or their component parts (e.g. diagnostic tests, treatments, caring procedures) fulfil stated goals' (St. Leger *et al.* 1992: 1). The increasing influence of evidence-based medicine on Department of Health thinking and policy making means that clinical practices are now being set against high standards of evaluation to assess whether they are cost-effective (Cochrane Database of Systematic Reviews 1996).

Participation of managers in evaluation is now starting to gain pace. In recent years there has been an explosion of interest in evidence-based medicine (EBM), and this is reflected in the development of systematic reviews, which are structured summaries of the results of research projects. The origins of EBM lie in the birth of randomized clinical trials and the increasing recognition of the importance of scientific evidence to guide the delivery of health care interventions.

This chapter will give mental health service managers an overview of why evaluation is important, the levels and phases of evaluation, the key features of evaluation measures and the main methods of evaluation. It will also guide managers to the sources of research findings by giving an extended section on further reading, with some simple examples of how to get started on your own service evaluation.

Why evaluate?

Evaluation is necessary to establish whether a service achieves its goals. This implies that service goals are explicitly stated. Some of the advantages for managers of commissioning or attending to evaluation are shown in the following list. It is also important for managers to know if the effects of their services are consistent with national policy. The reasons for evaluation are:

- to assess which services are achieving defined goals and which are not
- to support decisions for service development, decommissioning or changes
- to identify which service components to challenge for evidence
- to establish if initial start-up investment should be continued as revenue
- to use as a negotiation tool for purchasers or providers
- to form a basis for discussion with clinicians on quality of service.

It is important to understand three key 'Es' – efficacy, effectiveness and efficiency – as the goals of evaluation. By *efficacy* we mean the therapeutic potential of a treatment, in other words how far it improves outcomes under ideal experimental conditions. By comparison, clinical *effectiveness* can be defined as the actual results obtained by an intervention in routine patient populations who seek care from routine clinical services. *Effectiveness* can be defined at the service user level as 'the proven, intended benefits of treatments provided in real-life situations', or it can be defined at the local service level as 'the proven, intended benefits of services provided in real life situations' (Thornicroft and Tansella 1999). By comparison we define *efficiency*, as used within health economics, as 'a service characteristic, which minimizes the inputs needed to achieve a given level of outcomes, or which maximizes the outcomes for a given level of inputs'. Efficiency is therefore a combination of effectiveness and costs, or in other words, the relationship between inputs and outputs. Effectiveness is related to efficiency, and Cochrane and Bal (1977) have stressed the primacy of effectiveness for attaining efficiency. As Light (1991) has put it, 'can one increase efficiency through competitive contracts if the contractors do not know what is effective?' Indeed, Light (1991) has reinterpreted Cochrane's classic work to produce what he calls the 'Cochrane test', which summarizes many of the aims of health service evaluation. The central point is that what matters is what objective you have established. Within this context, how many mental health services can pass these six central and pragmatic effectiveness questions?

1 Consider anything that works.
2 Make effective treatments available to all.
3 Minimize ill time interventions.
4 Treat service users in the most effective place.
5 Prevent only what is preventable.
6 Diagnose only if treatable.

Evaluation levels and phases

Before looking at the more technical aspects of evaluation we shall offer a framework called the matrix model (Thornicroft and Tansella 1999), to act as a map to understand where different types of evaluation take place. The two dimensions of this conceptual framework are the geographical and the temporal (see Table 8.1). The first of these refers to three *geographical* levels: (1) country, (2) local and (3) service user. The second dimension refers to three *temporal* levels: (A) inputs, (B) processes and (C) outcomes. Using these two dimensions we construct a 3 × 3 matrix to bring into focus critical issues for mental health services.

Evaluation can take place in any of the cells of the matrix model. We believe that the primary purpose of mental health services is to optimize individual outcomes (cell 3C). It is notable that many types of service assessment, audit and evaluation take place at almost every other cell and are interpreted *as if* they are associated with better service user outcomes.

Table 8.1   Overview of the matrix model, with examples of key issues in each cell of the matrix

Temporal dimension

		A Input phase	B Process phase	C Outcome phase
Geographical dimension	1 Country/ regional level	1A e.g. expenditure on services	1B e.g. performance/ activity indicators such as admission rates	1C e.g. suicide rates
	2 Local level (catchment area)	2A e.g. staff resources	2B e.g. caseloads	2C e.g. outcomes of groups of service users
	3 Service user level	3A e.g. individual treatments	3B e.g. continuity of care	3C e.g. symptom levels or satisfaction

For example, government may increase financial investment in the services as a whole (national input, cell 1A) and suggest that this will have a positive effect on service users. Equally, a local catchment area service may decrease the waiting time from GP referral to first out-patient assessment appointment (a local level process change) and again interpret this as an improvement, without also evaluating whether this has any effect upon service user outcomes.

Given this degree of confusion it is important to be clear about the meanings of key terms. We first therefore define as *inputs* 'the resources which are put into the mental health care system' (definitions from Thornicroft and Tansella 1998). The categories of inputs to mental health services are:

Budget
• absolute amount of money allocated to mental health services
• proportionate allocation in relation to total health expenditure or other indicators.

Staff
• numbers of staff at each level
• mix of professions.

Policies and regulations
- laws
- service standards
- treatment protocols and guidelines.

Media representations of mental health issues

Equipment and technology for investigation, diagnosis and treatment

Public attitudes to mental health issues

Buildings and facilities

Second, we define as *process* 'those activities which take place to deliver mental health services'. Many of these processes form the data that mental health services managers have regular access to. In terms of evaluation, a number of variables are commonly used to reflect these processes that refer to cell 2B of the matrix model. The definitions of variables (from Gater *et al.* 1995) that may be used to describe the process of care at the local level are:

- annual treated incidence
- annual treated prevalence
- one-day treated prevalence
- long-term service users on one day.
- in-patient prevalence
- total admissions
- first ever admissions
- readmissions
- mean number of beds occupied per day
- mean length of stay
- admission rates for service users in contact with services
- in-patient care priority index for specific diagnostic groups.
- day hospital prevalence
- mean day hospital contacts
- day hospital care priority index for specific diagnostic groups.
- out-patient and casual contact prevalence
- mean out-patients and casual contact
- out-patients priority index for specific diagnostic groups.
- home visits and community contacts prevalence
- mean home visits and community contacts
- home visits priority index for specific diagnostic groups.

Processes can also be evaluated at the national level (cell 1B), and one set of relevant data in the UK is the health service indicators published annually by the Department of Health. Glover (1996) gives these examples of mental health variables included in UK health service indicators:

- mental illness episodes that started within the year, where residents are not treated within district
- percentage of residents who are compulsorily detained in hospital
- ratio of first admissions for residents aged 75+ to total population of that age group
- percentage of admitted patients who are compulsorily admitted to hospital
- percentage of admitted service users who are compulsorily treated in hospital
- admission rate to mental health facilities per 100,000 total population
- number of compulsory hospital admissions per 10,000 total population
- percentage of all admissions that are first ever admissions
- first contact by community psychiatric nurses per 1,000 total population by age.

Third, *outcome* is defined in the *Concise Oxford Dictionary* as 'a result, a visible effect'. This sense that an outcome is the final step of a sequence of events is reinforced by the synonyms given for *outcome* in the *Oxford Thesaurus*, which include 'decision, determination, effect, end, event, fate, fruit, issue, judgement, pay-off, product, purpose, repercussion, resolution, result, solution, and upshot'. At the level of individual service users, which in our view should be the final common point towards which all service interventions are targeted, a number of evaluation domains are common to assess outcomes. These are:

- symptom severity
- service satisfaction
- quality of life
- disability
- impact on care-givers
- met and unmet needs.

In another sense, whole local services can be evaluated, either by formal research projects or by detailed inquiries. Most often this happens in practice only after a severe adverse event, and not as a matter of course. Important information can emerge from these reports, for example the themes emerging from a detailed analysis of recent evaluations of adverse events in London, as outlined below. Given the usefulness of the findings it is unfortunate that so much evaluation of mental health services occurs *after* a tragedy, rather than as part of the systematic and ongoing development and management of the local service. According Lelliot *et al.* (1997), the most common themes from special mental health service inquiries in London (in order of frequency) are:

- the adequacy and allocation of resources
- poor communication between agencies (especially between health and social services, between mental health and housing departments, and between specialist mental health services and GPs)

- poor assessment of the risk of violence
- problems in discharge of the patient from hospital (especially failure to assess needs and develop an aftercare plan)
- liaison with police and probation services
- confidentiality and professional ethics (especially as barriers between health and social services, and between mental health services and the police).

Key features of evaluation measures

At the individual service user level, researchers attach a high importance to the psychometric properties of the evaluation measures they use. First, they want to know if the 'instruments' (i.e. measurement scales) are *valid*: do they actually measure what they are intended to measure. Second, they assess if each scale is *reliable*: can it be used consistently by several raters, or at more than one time point; in other words, does it give repeatable results for the same service user when used under different conditions. In terms of formal research, the use of an evaluation scale that is not valid and reliable can seriously weaken the results (Thornicroft and Tansella 1996). So, it is always important to question research and the data generated to ensure that it is both valid and reliable before value is attached to the findings.

Evaluation methods

Evaluations may be classified as either *descriptive* or *analytical*. Descriptive studies seek to monitor the performance of a service at one time or over several time points. Comparisons can be *internal*, for instance comparing one aspect of the service against its performance at an earlier time, or *external*, in which the comparison is with other services or more widely validated standards. Analytical evaluations attempt to explain a process or outcome, for instance research projects that aim to identify the cause of a disease. In brief, it is often extraordinarily difficult to establish the causes of particular disorders, and in the mental health field it is often true that many causes acting at the same time influence the onset and course of a condition.

Any association found by research may or may not be causal. A leading British epidemiologist, Sir Austin Bradford Hill, has proposed nine criteria by which any pattern of associations (correlations between two variables) can be assessed for its likelihood of being of causal importance, namely: strength of the association, consistency, specificity, temporality, biological, gradient, plausibility, coherence, and experimental evidence (Hill 1965). These factors therefore need to be kept in mind when considering whether a correlation between two variables, for example the creation of a new community mental health team and a change in bed occupancy rates, is causally related or not.

Evaluation designs

For the sake of clarity we can distinguish four types of evaluation commonly found in mental health services research: Randomized Clinical Trials (RCT); Non-Randomized Clinical Trials (quasi-experimental studies, NRCT); Structured Clinical Practice (routine outcome studies, SCP); and Unstructured Clinical Practice (UCP). This classification acknowledges the importance of information gathered from RCTs, and also offers a context in which some value can be attached to Structured Clinical Practice to address questions for which randomized and non-randomized clinical trials are too costly or too premature. At the level of individual service user outcome research, the preferred direction for research design for therapeutic interventions should be from Unstructured Clinical Practice to Randomized Clinical Trials, and may pass through the intermediate stages of Structured Clinical Practice and Non-Randomized Clinical Trials.

Sources of evaluation findings

Most research work is entirely unknown to those who could benefit from it or to those who make decisions concerning the provision and structure of services. It is therefore important to know how to access the results of evaluative work to help you to do your job. Some useful sources of evaluation information are:

Written material (from librarian or research and development officer)
- academic journals for primary research (e.g. *British Journal of Psychiatry*)
- review journals for secondary analyses of findings (e.g. *Current Opinion in Psychiatry, Bombardier, Effectiveness Bulletin*)
- professional publications (e.g. *Health Service Journal*)
- occasional reports (e.g. Audit Commission)
- results of external evaluation (e.g. audits, benchmarking accreditation, and specific inquiries).

Electronic material (from IT department or colleague with IT skills)
- remote databases (e.g. Medline, Embase, Psychlit)
- WWW pages, using a search program for key words
- Cochrane database of systematic reviews.

Personal contact (from colleagues and/or allies)
- local librarian
- information officer of your local agencies
- public health physicians
- phone contact with colleagues
- information from conferences
- service user satisfaction surveys
- site visits to similar services
- clinicians working with you

- chief executive's office
- director of nursing.

Commencing evaluation within your service area

While we have outlined the basis of more formal evaluation methods in this chapter, we would encourage you to apply simple, structured approaches to many aspects of your managerial work. For example, for a new out-of-hours service, it will be important for you and your clinical colleagues to record the numbers of referrals, the sources, the types and place of assessments, and the ongoing treatment plans made for the cases seen. You may initially not be confident about how to establish a structured method, and in this case the following sources of support may be available: local audit staff, the Public Health Department of the health authority, local academic departments, staff within your team or service who have undertaken a formal academic training, or staff at the Research and Development Directorate of your health region.

Surviving jargon

Medical and health services research are clouded by jargon that tends to leave the non-expert mystified. We give some common jargon in mental health services research in the Jargon box.

References and further reading

Bowling, A. (1997) *Research Methods in Health. Investigating Health and Health Services*. Buckingham: Open University Press.

Cochrane, A. and Bal, J. (1977) Mental illness in immigrants to England and Wales: an analysis of mental hospital admissions, 1971, *Social Psychiatry*, 12: 25–35.

Cochrane Database of Systematic Reviews (1996) in The Cochrane Library [database on disk and CD-ROM]. Oxford: The Cochrane Collaboration. Software updated quarterly. Available from: BMJ Publishing Group, London.

Gater, R., Amaddeo, F., Tansella, M., Jackson, G. and Goldberg, D. (1995) A comparison of community based care for schizophrenia in South Verona and South Manchester, *British Journal of Psychiatry*, 166: 344–52.

Glover, G. (1996) Health service indictors for mental health, in G. Thornicroft and G. Strathdee (eds) *Commissioning Mental Health Services*, Appendix 311–18. London: HMSO.

Hill, A.B. (1965) The environment and disease: association or causation? *Proceedings of the Royal Society of Medicine*, 295–300.

Knudsen, H.C. and Thornicroft, G. (1996) *Mental Health Service Evaluation*. Cambridge: Cambridge University Press.

Lelliot, P., Audini, P., Johnson, S. and Guite, H. (1997) London in the context of mental health policy, in S. Johnson, L. Brooks, G. Thornicroft, L. Brooks, P. Lelliot, E. Peck, H. Smith, D. Chisholm, B. Audini, M. Knapp and D. Goldberg (eds) *London's Mental Health*. London: King's Fund.

Jargon box

audit the systematic, critical analysis of the quality of care, including the procedures used for diagnosis and treatment, the use of resources, and the resulting outcome and quality of life for the service user

dissemination the distribution of knowledge to those in a position to benefit from it

effectiveness the actual results obtained by an intervention in unselected service user populations who seek care from routine clinical services. In other words, the extent to which outcomes meet objectives

efficacy the therapeutic potential of a treatment, i.e. how far it improves outcomes under optimal experimental conditions

efficiency a service characteristic that maximizes outputs for a given input

evidence-based medicine a clinical practice that uses techniques shown by research to be effective

instrument a measurement scale used in research

intervention study a research project in which a specific treatment is offered to a group of service users and in which the status of the service users is evaluated before and after the intervention to measure the treatment effect

meta-analysis a technique used in evidence-based medicine in which the results of a series of research studies (usually randomized controlled trials) are examined in a highly structured way (a systematic review) to look for patterns in the results

subject a service user in a research study

randomized controlled trial a type of research study design in which a group of service users is randomly allocated into two or more groups to receive a new treatment or comparison treatments (conditions) and in which their status is evaluated before and after treatment to measure any treatment outcomes

---

Light, D.W. (1991) Effectiveness and efficiency under competition: the Cochrane test, *British Medical Journal*, 303: 1253–4.

Ong, B. (1993) *The Practice of Health Services Research*. London: Chapman and Hall.

St. Leger, A., Schneiden, H. and Walsworth-Bell, J. (1992) *Evaluating Health Services' Effectiveness*. Buckingham: Open University Press.

Thompson, C. (1989) *The Instruments of Psychiatric Research*. Chichester: Wiley.

Thornicroft, G. and Tansella, M. (eds) (1996) *Mental Health Outcome Measures*. Heidelberg: Springer Verlag.

Thornicroft, G. and Tansella, M. (1998) *The Mental Health Matrix*. Cambridge: Cambridge University Press.

Wetzler, S. (1989) *Measuring Mental Illness*. Washington, DC: American Psychiatry Press.

Section C
The six key managerial tasks

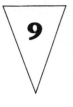

9 | Task 1 Managing the change process

Key themes

In this chapter we aim to help you:

- understand how change affects individuals and organizations
- spot the pitfalls associated with change
- prepare for change
- motivate staff to accept change
- manage anxiety and opposition to change
- break change down into achievable tasks
- provide ways to create certainty when all is changing.

Changes therefore need to be planned and managed since the effective operation of a complex service demands the goodwill, competence and co-operation *of its staff.*
(Glynn and Perkins, *Managing Health Care – Challenges for the 90s* 1995: 115)

Introduction

There was a time when large organizations (particularly hospitals and health care providers) remained stable and predictable places to work. Changes would come at intervals, be time-limited and all would return to relative normality after the change had occurred. In the last decade major changes have occurred in the NHS at every level, and as a result, change is now the norm and the predictable is the exception. This means that the ability to bring about and successfully achieve change is a key skill for all managers, and therefore we can expect to be involved in and leading change programmes as part of the normal course of our future working lives.

This chapter looks at change in more detail, and offers some guidance *on how to approach change*, based on our own experiences and those of colleagues across the UK. We have concentrated on three areas of a complex change process: getting started, taking people with you and communicating well. While the examples are taken from major hospital reprovision programmes that we or colleagues have been involved in, the themes could also apply to other types of change management. You may, for example, find yourself developing an out-of-hours service, or a specialist out-patient provision. In each case, good planning, motivation of others and a clear communication stream will be vital. Our focus here is on the practical aspects of change, rather than on the theory of change management, which is already plentiful. We shall use case studies to illustrate some of the key issues likely to be encountered when planning and implementing changes in mental health services. We have deliberately focused on topics within such change programmes that we think will be relevant to mental health service providers elsewhere.

Our three *case studies* refer to examples of the management processes involved in (i) project-managing moving acute psychiatric beds from an old institutional setting to a newly developed unit at a different site, and (ii) overcoming staff resistance during a change programme. The first case study examines the *initiation stage*, and includes a discussion of the project manager's role, how to structure the necessary meetings, and how to include and motivate clinical staff in the process.

Our second case example will describe our experience of how to manage the inevitable staff reactions of *resistance*, *anxiety* and *concerns* associated with change, and reflects upon the predictable need to resolve these reactions positively if the project is to succeed.

Case study 3 focuses on the necessary infrastructure elements that will be required to *communicate* with staff during the service development process, and the ongoing communication needs of staff when the *consolidation* stage begins to take place.

Case study 1 Preparing for change and avoiding the pitfalls

Our first case study refers to the earliest stages of an acute in-patient bed reprovision programme. One key lesson that we have learned from such a change is that careful and detailed planning is vital for a successful outcome. This can often feel tedious, and many managers are tempted to jump in and get on with things. This is something both of us have mistakenly done, particularly when working to tight time-frames. While careful and detailed planning is crucial, we do not necessarily mean lengthy planning cycles, endless meetings, gant charts and repeated discussions. While all of these have their place, it is important not to get caught up solely in the process, as this is not the aim. We refer instead to real, pragmatic and considered planning. This planning should prepare sufficiently for the change, but it should also recognize the importance of taking the staff with you. Mental health services (perhaps more than other areas of the health care system) rely primarily on the skills of clinicians to deliver effective treatments to service users. Therefore, poorly informed and potentially resistant staff will not assist an effective programme of change.

Your approach needs to be flexible enough to adapt itself during the service transition. Delays in such processes are very frequent and should not be feared, but they should be used constructively. We all hope that change is straightforward and goes exactly as planned, but we have never yet encountered such a project!

Our starting point for this case study is the appointment of a project manager to lead a hospital reprovision programme. The project manager reported directly to the Trust directors and was given overall responsibility for the closure of the large institution and the move of staff and service users into the new service. This included overseeing the building programme, preparing staff for the move, developing operational procedures for the new services and coordinating the communication and involvement of Trust staff throughout the change process.

Because these were the first major service moves that the Trust had undertaken since its inception, there was a general underestimation of the scale of the change that had been taken on, and the complexities of the tasks involved. The appointment of one person to coordinate such diverse and demanding responsibilities was therefore not realistic.

Comment

It would have been useful at the earliest stage to have developed a project group representing all the task areas rather than appoint one person to do everything. If such a team still does not include some key skills, one option is then to redeploy or co-opt key members of staff from elsewhere within your organization, or from local partner organizations, on a part-time or short-term basis. Where this is still insufficient, a second option is to recruit such skills in from outside. This process requires a specific brief for each project on the core key skills necessary for the project group to meet its targets.

Soon after appointment the project manager established a planning team for each of the component moves within the whole project. The meetings of the team were chaired by the project manager. It was comprised of representatives from each ward and department as well as operational managers and the Trust's Facilities Manager. In addition, service user representatives were invited to attend so that their views could be incorporated into the overall planning process.

The membership of the group soon appeared to be too fluid; bringing staff and representatives from many different levels of the organization together did not achieve the clarity of purpose and direction the group needed, often best stated as a written set of terms of reference for each individual meeting. The clinical services moving into the new building had different needs, and this was often frustrating as these conflicts dominated the meeting and other services did not get their concerns adequately addressed. To many in the group the move seemed too far off and too remote to concern them. An important point here is that clinicians, trained in short-term treatments, are generally not used to working to two- or three-year timeframes in the same way as project managers. The change process therefore needs to be brought closer to them and made relevant:

> One of the methods devised for achieving quick action is what Peters and Waterman term 'chunking'. Chunking is an approach whereby a problem that arises in an organisation is first made manageable (i.e. broken into chunks) and then tackled by a small group of staff brought together specifically for that purpose.
>
> (Burns 1992: 58)

Membership of the project group was becoming irregular and inefficient, and as the ward move dates became closer, the project manager realized that the project was not on course. He therefore instigated a sub-group structure for the project group. This proved successful because people were invited to attend a particular interest group and then to report back to the commissioning team on progress. The groups devised at this stage concentrated on staffing changes, support services required and communication issues. Because these groups were tightly focused with clear objectives they worked well. The momentum for change began to develop after the introduction of 'chunking'.

Comment

The Trust realized that a successful change project needs to involve more than a few individuals. The involvement of staff and staff groups in the task groups was itself a trigger to getting the change programme started. This is reinforced by the view of Douglas Wallace, Vice President of Social Policy, North Western National Bank: 'Working with employees on task forces . . . is like watching a steam locomotive with a big load of cars begin to chug-a-chug. Eventually it gets such a head of steam that its momentum is difficult to slow down' (cited in Kanter 1983).

In *Managing Change* Bernard Burns (1992) has stated some important characteristics of successful task groups. You may wish to use this as a checklist for your own project. Task groups:

- usually comprise no more than ten members
- are voluntarily constituted
- have a life of usually between three and six months
- have a membership whose reporting level/seniority is appropriate to the problem

- document their proceedings informally and minimally
- have a limited set of objectives, determined and monitored by the group.

We have found that with complex change programmes it is important to clarify the group structure and reporting arrangements as soon as possible. Some of the structural characteristics of a successful planning group are:

- there is also an information sharing/feedback group
- there are small task groups, with agreed membership and clear time limits
- strong chairing of the feedback group helps monitor progress of task groups
- members are willing to concentrate on process not structures
- there is a fixed and committed core membership
- the feedback group is comprised of both visionaries and strategists
- the task groups are made up of 'doers' and action-orientated people.

Planning in the task groups of this reprovision programme initially progressed well, but after one year the project suffered a major setback. The building contractors went into liquidation and an inevitable and unsettling delay ensued. The contract for building works was speedily retendered but it soon became clear that the original project completion date would not be achieved.

This delay caused a great deal of uncertainty and disappointment for staff at all levels in the organization. The result was that suspicion about the reliability of the move dates and timescales dogged the rest of the project, and the distrust needed active work by managers in order to maintain morale. Nevertheless, there were also benefits resulting from the delay. Around the time that the contractors pulled out the project team were becoming increasingly aware of the complexities involved in the physical moves of the services, staff and service users. Prior to this all of the energies had been concentrated on designing and equipping the buildings. The five-month delay therefore became a vital period during which the detail of organizational change and the preparation of staff for the changes took place. In hindsight, had the team not had the delay the services would not have moved as effectively and smoothly as they eventually did.

In summary, this first case study has been used to highlight some of the important factors to consider when commencing a change programme within your own organization. We have also attempted to reinforce the need for a planned and reflective approach throughout any change planning phase. We also learned that improvements and better solutions do sometimes arise from setbacks and delays. Handling delays and disappointments is difficult; we may feel that our reputation is at stake, along with the expectations and hopes of our staff. If we are to be effective and respected managers then setbacks can provide useful if unwelcome occasions for learning. Do not get sidetracked in the disappointments or delays.

Use the opportunity to reflect, take stock and plan for when things start moving again. The following list is a summary of some of the common pitfalls that are illustrated by this first case study:

- underestimation of the importance of thorough planning
- not devising a team to manage the change process
- appointing a change manager to tackle everything!
- unrealistic timescales
- not using setbacks constructively
- not persuading staff of the rationale for change
- staff feeling that change is being imposed
- suspicions about the 'real' reasons for change
- insufficient time invested in working with staff at each stage
- having more 'visionaries' than 'doers' in the task groups
- lack of trust and confidence in change leaders from the clinical staff.

Case study 2 Motivating staff to accept change

The important point to remember is that if you are trying to motivate someone else, you must consider what it is that motivates them and not what would motivate you in similar circumstances . . . If we start by thinking about them, and what enthuses them and what irritates them (without making judgements, just recognising differences) we can avoid this.

(Iles 1997: 11)

Our second case example is an illustration of how staff initially opposed a service change. It offers suggestions on how *to understand the context and reasons for such resistance*, and then how to deal with it constructively.

In terms of the background to this case study, during the few months immediately prior to the relocation of a psychiatric in-patient service, there had been several unpleasant assaults by service users on staff, some of whom had been seriously injured. There had been some long-standing opinions among the ward nursing staff that the planned new ward building was not suitable for its use as a mental health unit, and following these incidents some staff became even more concerned about their safety. A few members of staff vehemently expressed their opinion that the new building would be dangerous because direct observation of service users would be difficult, as there were many blind spots. However, their main area of concern focused upon the reliability of the wall-mounted violence alarm system that was being installed. Ward staff had previously been using a hand-held radio-controlled system and felt that the new alarm system was less safe. The alarm system had become the main topic of conversation among staff at nearly every nurse staff meeting in the few months before the relocation. As this date approached, from a managerial perspective it became imperative that this issue was resolved effectively, and it required sensitive handling so that staff anxieties were diminished.

Such anxieties are to be expected, and in fact are reasonable reactions to unpredictability. Staff will always have mixed feelings about imminent changes, and these concerns may become fixed on new physical structures, such as the alarm system, or upon more clinical topics, such as the types of service users to be treated in different ward areas. At the same time, some staff will appreciate early on the positive impact that the new facilities can have for service users and staff, with improved accommodation and a better working environment. The careful manager will need to predict such staff feelings, and can minimize their extent by offering clear information at each stage of the transition, by making sure that staff have time to talk to middle managers, who do listen to their anxieties, and by altering physical structures and operational policies to make material changes, as far as possible, to reassure staff.

Factors in the local and national political context can also shape the nature and scale of these concerns. For example, developing a new community mental health team at the time of a local public inquiry into a high profile homicide may unnerve staff. Similarly, a relatively common occurrence is for service changes to be proposed at the same time that cuts in clinical budgets are being implemented, which may be two entirely separate developments. Clinical staff may reasonably conclude that the service changes are only motivated by cost-cutting. The service development may therefore founder unless skilfully handled by managers who understand the relevance of the local and national contexts, and who are able to persuade staff – if this is actually the case – that the two sets of initiatives are separate. The main point is that managers need to understand what is uppermost in the minds of clinical staff and to appreciate their usually legitimate multiple motivations, in order to be successful in persuading them that service changes are genuinely intended to offer benefits to service users.

Comment

The alarm system and its safety was of genuine concern to the staff. Yet, the mounting strength of staff feelings surprised managers. On reflection, the alarm system appeared to have become the main single focus for many different anxieties about the change process itself.

John Van Maurik in his book *Discovering the Leader in You* (1994) describes some common reasons why people are often reluctant to accept change. Staff may:

- feel left in the dark
- not feel consulted about the change
- feel threatened and a pawn in the game
- not understand what is proposed
- consider that other options are better
- think change is unnecessary.

In response to staff concerns, and in an attempt to manage these fears, ward staff were invited by managers to walk around the new building, to describe their concerns and their reasons in more detail, and to test out the new alarm system by going through simulations of real emergencies. Although some managers argued that such involvement would produce unnecessary delays and costs, and actually reinforce staff anxieties, the prevailing view was that direct care staff do have invaluable insights into the clinical consequences of the ward layout, and may help to avoid bad decisions being put into practice. At the same time, if staff do not feel closely involved from the outset in such a process, they will eventually slow the whole implementation process down even more by continuing to raise objections at any later stage. One of the key managerial skills here is to listen to suggestions and to be able to separate constructive proposals (those that are both feasible and will contribute towards a better quality of care), from those perhaps better seen as indirect expressions of 'change anxiety'.

Prior to walking around the ward with clinical staff, the managerial view, based on drawings of the system, was that the alarms were adequate. In fact, direct observation blind spots were identified in some of the wards, along with the need for more alarm points, and it was agreed with staff that these problems would be rectified before the ward moves went ahead. Engaging with the clinical staff therefore helped the managers to appreciate the issues more closely, and to find acceptable solutions.

Comment

Although the staff were not initially happy to change to wall mounted violence alarms, these timely actions by managers greatly relieved the anxieties of staff, most of whom felt that their concerns had been both listened to and responded to. This intervention was a demonstration that managers were not just imposing change, but were also trying to take staff with them in the process.

In reviewing this case study there are some key lessons when facing staff resistance or opposition to change programmes:

- remember that change will produce anxieties; be prepared
- pre-empt possible anxiety-provoking decisions
- plan a strategy to deal with resistance
- concerns expressed by staff are real to them (if not to you)
- explain changes (especially unpopular ones) in relation to service user benefit
- explain the rationale many times – anxious people do not listen carefully
- use influential staff wisely to disseminate the reasons for change
- face-to-face meetings with clear agendas are usually more effective for dealing with anxieties
- never only communicate unpopular decisions or major changes in writing.

It is worth reflecting on the variety of qualities required by managers during such a process. Indeed, there are several paradoxes for a manager that appear throughout any change project. The first paradox is that the manager is required to show enthusiasm for the project, yet at the same time to balance this with sensitivity towards the staff involved. The enthusiasm on the part of the manager will generate dedication to see the project through. This, if not tempered, can become overwhelming and even more anxiety-provoking for staff. It is important therefore to use one's own enthusiasm to encourage and develop confidence in the project for the more reluctant staff.

The second paradox is that the manager needs to demonstrate both toughness and gentleness in approach. The toughness is necessary to make important and difficult decisions that will keep the project moving ahead, while retaining a gentleness of style that will accept constructive criticism and overcome disappointments along the way. Without such gentleness the manager can be perceived as dictatorial and will not win vital organizational support.

The third paradox for the manager is that between tenacity and flexibility. The manager must show determination in sticking with a process, even when things are at their most difficult. Taken to extreme, this trait can become unyielding without sufficient flexibility. The contrast here is between a determination to achieve the longer-term objective of a project, with a high degree of willingness by the manager to be flexible in incorporating shorter-term and unplanned variations (which will be specific to each local situation) on how best to reach the project goal.

Case study 3   Creating routine infrastructure during a change process

Our third case study illustrates the importance of using two types of infrastructure, within which the uncertainties of change can be made manageable: (i) clear and systematic forms of communication, and (ii) predictable operational routines.

In terms of communication, our first theme, one of the most frustrating experiences we have had, in service development projects, was hearing the phrase 'I never knew about that'. In one particular project, the creation of a new mental health day centre in South London, as the day of opening came closer, decisions were being made quickly as planning meetings tended to take more and more of staff time. At such critical periods, managers will tend to concentrate on operational matters rather than continue to keep all staff informed of the decisions that have been made. It is common just before completion of such projects for an information gap to open up in which the majority of staff may be several months out of date in the information available to them, and an initial consensus can deteriorate over time. As recipients of organizational news, all managers appreciate the need to communicate information quickly and effectively, but they may not also sufficiently recognize their role as information providers, especially to operational clinical and administrative staff.

A number of meetings may be useful. These can provide the infrastructure necessary to manage the wide range of necessary functions and can establish a framework of regular and stable predictability, both to keep staff updated and actively to manage the need for reassurance. In the case of the completion of the new day centre, we used the following methods:

1 A regular management team meeting was set up, that began at monthly intervals and became, for a fixed period of three months, weekly to manage the amount of business that we needed to transact. Its role was to:
   - take key decisions
   - coordinate communication to staff
   - synchronize all aspects of the project
   - cascade information to regular staff meetings for the sector service
   - invite other key parties as required, especially the works department, press department and non-clinical support service managers.
2 A monthly communications group oversaw briefings, and sent out a regular newsletter to:
   - service users, relatives and other carers
   - neighbours
   - other departments within the provider Trust
   - outside agencies, including police, social services and voluntary groups.
3 Informal face-to-face meetings with staff, service users and other parties were useful in:
   - conveying the latest information
   - answering questions
   - helping to assess the adequacy of communication flows.
4 A daily clinical meeting was started for all clinical staff in the community mental health team and day centre staff (from 9.00 to 9.15 a.m.). This morning clinical meeting was started before the clinical teams moved into their new premises, and it served as a source of predictable stability and an opportunity to speak to other members of staff for non-urgent matters. This meeting acted in the following ways:
   - staff could be updated on important clinical issues arising since the previous meeting
   - it enabled staff to report admissions and status of in-patients from the sector
   - urgent visits or assessments that were pending could be allocated
   - cover for unplanned leave or absence could be arranged
   - it helped to introduce visitors and new staff
   - staff could be alerted to service users who were relapsing or who were causing other concern
   - it provided a forum for the announcing of the duty medical, nursing and social work staff for the day.

Comment

It is important to remember that change removes routine, structure and order, which are important for individuals and for teams. Change always produces anxiety in individuals, and this anxiety creates a temporary need for even more structure than in times of greater stability. It is important not to underestimate the need for regular, routine meetings, information circulars and channels of communication. These can be pre-existing structures that develop a new importance, and perhaps a greater frequency during a transitional period, or new forums that become important for the duration of the change.

One very useful channel developed for communication with staff during a change programme is the team briefing note. In the example of the new day centre, following the operational team meeting a monthly briefing note was devised and circulated to all day centre staff involved directly in the service changes, to members of the local community mental health team, and to Trust central departments. The content of the briefing was all decisions made in the preceding month, any other news relating to the move, and to feed back particular information in response to questions from staff. It was useful for quashing untrue rumours that were circulating swiftly around the organization as the change programme gained pace. Some of the key points to remember in a team briefing note are:

- be clear about the purpose of the briefing note (information sharing or to involve in decision making)
- state on the briefing note who is the author
- state who the note is being circulated to
- date the document so staff will then know how recent the information is
- list decisions that have been made and those still to be taken
- make it eye-catching, e.g. use coloured paper, a logo or bold heading
- say how staff can contribute to the briefing note
- use briefing notes to remind staff of key dates and events
- try to incorporate some fun items – this may get staff interested
- edit/proof-read for jargon and relevance before circulating!

Before deciding how best to provide communication channels within your own organization, it may be helpful to undertake a simple communication audit. This will identify areas of weakness. Perhaps there may be poor communication in your own team or organization because you:

- make false assumptions
- tell people what *you* think they need to hear rather than what *they* say they want to hear
- assume staff read papers circulated to them
- give key information only once rather than enough times
- think what is important to you is also important to others
- forget that anxiety clogs the mind

- do not reinforce written communication with face-to-face contact
- do not have a high profile – not enough face-to-face meetings.

The communication audit will suggest options to help devise an action plan for improved communication.

Conclusion

In using these three case studies we have sought to outline some of the key factors vital to a successful change project. These can be summarized (based on Kanter 1983) as:

- change requires stability
- change requires energy
- change requires time
- change requires commitment
- change needs continuity of key people
- change requires a measure of security.

References and further reading

Burns, B. (1992) *Managing Change*. London: Pitman Publishing.

Glynn, J. and Perkins, A. (1995) *Managing Health Care – Challenges for the 90s*. Philadelphia: W.B. Saunders.

Iles, V. (1997) *Really Managing Health Care*. Buckingham: Open University Press.

Kanter, R.M. (1983) *The Change Masters – Corporate Entrepreneurs at Work*. London: Routledge.

Peters, T.J. and Waterman, R.H. (1989) *In Search of Excellence*. London: Harper-Collins.

Van Maurik, J. (1994) *Discovering the Leader in You*. New York: McGraw Hill.

Task 2 **The central role of human resources**

Key themes

In this chapter we aim to help you learn about:

- strategies for successful recruitment
- specifying job roles and developing staff
- flexibility in employment
- managing staff that struggle
- the importance of supervision.

Stress can be good, stress can be bad.
(Charles Handy, *Understanding Organisations* 1976)

Introduction

Our main theme in this chapter is the question: how can the human resources in any existing mental health service best be deployed for the benefit of service users? We shall not discuss basic human resource matters, which many readers are already familiar with. Instead we shall concentrate upon more pragmatic and day-to-day issues, and in effect we shall base our comments upon the evidence of our experience, rather than the evidence of research. This is simply because there is a striking absence of relevant research in this area.

To a greater extent than most other areas of medicine, mental health services rely upon human technology rather than upon instrumental technology, both for diagnosis and for therapy. In terms of treatments, it is clear

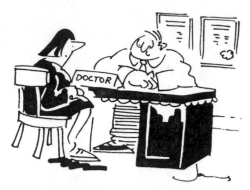

'You've got Scarlet Fever – and, frankly, my dear,
I don't give a damn'

that the human factor is central in how far, for example, service users comply with prescribed medication. Indeed it is within mental health services that the importance of the relationship between clinician and service user is most accentuated.

There are vital implications for this central role of the human factor. Apart from capital (buildings) costs, recurrent expenditure in mental health services is almost entirely used for the development and maintenance of human resources. Also the nature of clinical contact with psychiatric service users puts demands upon staff that draw upon all their reserves, and renders staff at risk of a depletion of motivation and compassion, the so-called 'burnout syndrome'. These human resources are therefore not fixed resources, but are continually subject to deterioration or degradation unless restored and upgraded.

From the outset we want to make the distinction between *primary* and *secondary* service goals. By primary goals we refer to interventions intended to give treatment, care and assistance to service users. In our view this is the central purpose of the service and should always remain centre-stage. By secondary goals we mean measures that are addressed to the needs of staff. Although in this chapter we shall argue that the quality of service to service users will suffer unless these necessary and legitimate staff needs are properly addressed, nevertheless within a wider context we continue to give primacy to service users' needs over those of staff. Indeed, when clinical teams can select only desirable service users (and exclude service users who are less rewarding or attractive), then service users' needs may become subsidiary to those of staff.

In this chapter we shall consider the management of human resources at the individual level. We shall go on to consider issues relevant to the team and to team management in Chapter 12. Although there are many books on the training of psychiatrists and other members of the mental health team, especially in relation to specific techniques for assessment and treatment, the question of how staff can be managed and developed in the wider perspective of a community-orientated service has received remarkably little attention.

When considering the staffing of mental health services several factors are worth noting. There is a need to consider personality and attitudinal factors in staff as individuals and as members of the team. This is particularly important when selecting new staff. The next stage is to acquire expertise, which has to be differentiated from experience.

Experience is simply directly proportional to the period of time spent on a particular task, without reference to quality, and derives from *experientia*, meaning to try, without necessarily succeeding. Expertise, on the other hand, is the acquisition of knowledge and skill or judgement for a given purpose. While a certain degree of experience is necessary to establish expertise, it does not necessarily follow that experience *per se* leads to expertise. Indeed, it is worth remembering here that some long-term staff may have accumulated many years of adverse or irrelevant experience, such as the custodial practices of some clinical staff in poor-quality institutions. In other words, it is expertise rather than experience that counts. So how does a service manager or team leader ensure that they recruit and develop staff who have the right blend of personality, attitude, training and expertise to be effective mental health staff and provide the highest-quality interventions for service users?

In beginning to look at human resources in more detail we have used the following headings as the structure of this chapter:

1 stock-taking and forward planning
2 roles and job specifications
3 recruitment and selection
4 staff appraisal, development and training
5 the flexible and understanding employer
6 helping those who struggle
7 good practice in supervision
8 preventing burnout.

These sections cover the main practical stages of staff management that you may be asked to address when you come into a new post, or when reviewing an existing team or service.

Stock-taking and forward planning

In starting to take stock of the human resources available to you, for example in a community mental health team or for a psychiatric in-patient ward, you may need to consider the total number of posts, the professions in those posts, whether they are full-time or part-time (session contributions are especially common for doctors and psychologists), whether the posts are filled or not by substantive appointments, and if staff are away on maternity, secondment, training or sick leave.

A second set of issues, having made an inventory of names, is to examine the question: how long are they here for? For posts, you will need to distinguish between temporary, fixed-term and permanent positions. For individuals this means establishing the starting dates for each member of staff, their contract lengths, when they retire, and also, over a period of time, finding out how long they actually want to stay in their current post, in your organization, and in your local area.

At the next stage it will be important also to take stock of all the other human resources available to your team. These may include trainees, students, honorary appointments, volunteers, and sessional individual or group therapists.

After the 'head-count' stage, you will want to go on to the more important question of establishing the skills and grades of staff. This is likely to involve individual meetings with professional heads of staff, or in some cases with the individual members of staff themselves. The purposes of such a skill audit are to: (i) establish whether the skill mix available to the whole team is suitable for its purpose, and (ii) decide how far postholders operate to their full potential, and are they performing the best possible role in the team. The importance of this stage is that it needs to be set against a 'team specification' (the team equivalent of a person specification) to see how far the current staff team matches the services needed by service users served in your local catchment area.

All of the information outlined above should enable you to draft a staff plan. This may then become the blueprint that you refer to as posts become vacant in your team or new resources become available to the service. It is worth noting that no team we have come across to date (unless devised as part of a research service) has had the breadth of skills, professions or grades that the service might ideally require. The important principle is therefore to decide the ideal staffing profile for the team to move towards and then to incrementally change the mix and staffing of the team as opportunities arise through vacancies, retirements or secondments of staff. Many managers may be tempted to move quickly to recruit to a vacancy on the basis of the leaver's qualification or profession, rather than for the skills that the post actually requires.

Roles and job specifications

Once you have identified what resources you have to hand in terms of posts and employed staff, and you have gone on to draft your staffing plan, you may next want to turn to devising or revising the job descriptions needed to support these roles. The job description or specification will outline the technical skills, qualifications and experience required to undertake each role. Although this is usually formulated for new posts, it is in fact equally important for existing staff, to refocus their role, and to prioritize and control work demand. It also provides an opportunity to discuss how the job may have changed or developed since its inception.

Also important, but rarely considered, are the personality traits or attitude of the individual you are seeking to recruit. Personality characteristics and attitudes are important factors to consider, particularly when you have the opportunity to recruit to a new role in the team. We agree with the qualities Mosher and Burti (1994) have described as desirable and undesirable for community mental health staff:

Desirable characteristics
1 strong sense of self: comfort with uncertainty
2 open minded: accepting and non-judgemental
3 service-user-focused and non-intrusive
4 practical, problem-solving orientation
5 flexible
6 empathic
7 optimistic and supportive
8 gentle firmness
9 humorous
10 humble
11 thinks contextually.

Undesirable characteristics
1 the rescue fantasy
2 consistent distortion of information
3 pessimistic outlook
4 exploitative of service users for own needs
5 over-controlling and needing to do for others
6 suspicious and accusatory towards others.

While these characteristics sketch a desirable profile for mental health practitioners, quite often one finds staff who are unsuited to clinical work, but who nevertheless have direct care responsibilities. How one might deal with these issues will be considered in more detail in the 'Helping those who struggle' section later.

The person specification, if carefully designed, will enable the whole process of recruitment and selection to run more smoothly and prevent time being wasted on interviewing unsuitable and unappointable candidates. Once the post is recruited to the job description this then sets the scope of the role to be performed by the individual. It will also be an invaluable point of reference if the individual begins to struggle in the post.

To assist in devising a person specification and job description you may wish to consider using the Munro Fraser Five Fold Framework found in Sisson (1994). This is shown in Table 10.1.

As part of the design of the job specification it is important to clarify how these skills and competencies you have identified will be assessed. The assessment methods you employ may include the application form, interview, presentation and taking up references. It is also worth differentiating between essential and desirable characteristics that you are looking for. In

Table 10.1   Munro Fraser's Five Fold framework

1 Impact on others	Appearance, speech, manner, self-confidence
2 Acquired knowledge or qualifications	Education, training, work experience
3 Innate abilities	Speed of perception, special aptitudes
4 Motivation	Goals, consistency, initiative, practical effectiveness
5 Emotional adjustment	Ability to cope with stress, flexibility, outlook

order not to exclude interesting candidates who may be able to develop skills that they do not currently possess, you may wish to keep the list of essential skills relatively short.

For example, when selecting a project manager to establish the new facilities for a developing community-based mental health service we selected an applicant who had worked both in health and local authority settings, and who understood inter-agency working from direct personal experience, but who did not have an established traditional career pattern. In this case we rated ability and potential over experience. In another case, after establishing the new community mental health teams, we appointed a clinical manager for a local sector service. It was important to select a strong consolidating force, and we therefore prioritized in this appointment relevant nursing experience, and team support and development skills.

Recruitment and selection

In our view recruitment and selection for mental health services staff can be seen in two ways: traditional and customized. The *traditional* approach is to take an off-the-shelf job description, update it slightly and advertise in the professional journals. This sees new staff as almost interchangeable and uniform commodities, who make standard contributions to the organization. This method may be entirely appropriate and cost-effective for many posts. At the same time, this model is best fitted to a stable working environment, such as a well-established in-patient nursing team, or an existing community service.

Increasingly, however, mental health services are undergoing transformation, or are developing in specialized ways, often in challenging environments, that have not existed before. Under these circumstances, a *customized* recruitment approach is likely to be needed. Before appointing a project manager, for example, it may be necessary to consider the different skills the individual will be required to demonstrate and the work environments they will have been exposed to. It may be, for example, that the successful candidate will not have come from a traditional NHS career path, but instead will have a hybrid career track. Increasingly, mental health services are delivered through multi-agency and multi-professional collaboration, and an individual from a very traditional career path may find this work context particularly challenging. It is therefore important that these necessary characteristics are reflected in the person specification and job description, and then incorporated into the advertisement and where the advert is to be placed. It is worth consulting with colleagues in neighbouring organizations (statutory and voluntary) about where they have successfully advertised, particularly if you have been impressed with the calibre of their staff.

In terms of the content of the advertisement a number of issues are important. First, it is important to give a true impression of the work context and the likely degree of pressure and pace that the postholder will be expected to maintain. Second, we suggest that you look upon the exercise as one in which you are recruiting to your *future* organization and its needs, rather than your current organization. This implies that you have a clear view of how you want your team or organization to develop, and of how this post fits into the overall pattern of skills that you will need to assemble. Third, it will often be helpful to have a clear view of the stage of service development; for example, an initiator will be needed early in a planned change process, and a consolidator at a later stage when the key tasks are bedding-in and stabilizing the service. From our own experience, it may be necessary from time to time to delay reappointment, and to take time to reflect on whether that whole post is still necessary, or whether it should be continued but in a modified way. As services become more differentiated, and with more varied appointments to bring closer working between mental health services, local authorities and primary care, so we expect that the customized approach will become ever more common.

Your organization is likely to have a standard application form. In addition to this, for specific posts you may wish to ask for particular additional supporting information. For example, in trying to upgrade an intensive care ward in a difficult inner city catchment area, local managers asked applicants for the ward manager role to write a short statement in response to the proposition: 'The pressure on hospital beds in intensive care units allows them to provide little more than security and medication: discuss.' The written contributions of the applicants very clearly differentiated between those with traditional custodial views, and those who saw the opportunities for innovation. The candidates in the latter category were shortlisted!

In terms of shortlisting, you will need to decide whether to interview all those who meet the minimum criteria, or only those who appear, on paper, to be the strongest candidates. In favour of the latter approach are time pressures, and a wish to avoid wasting the time of the panel with weaker applicants. For example, in shortlisting applicants for a clinical psychology training scheme, there will usually be many more suitably qualified applicants than vacancies. In this case, it may well be unnecessary to interview all applicants, and a short-list of the best six would suffice.

Several points arise at interview. First, the questions asked will need to reflect the full range of qualities and responsibilities expected of the new postholder. For a 'traditional' post, a standard panel will be sufficient. For 'customized' posts, an appropriately customized panel may be vital. For example, an advocacy scheme coordinator is likely to have a strong service user voice represented. Second, keep in mind the need to distinguish between expertise and experience: the latter may not confer the former! Third, be ready not to appoint. Remember that it can take 20 minutes to recruit a new member of staff and 20 years to get rid of them! It is therefore usually better not to appoint an unsuitable candidate. Fourth, do not make an offer or confirm an appointment unless you have received satisfactory references. This should include satisfactory work performance and work attendance (avoid the brilliant candidate who is off sick half the time). We suggest that you develop a slightly critical and reserved approach, in which you accept that your first impressions or the face value of an application may be wrong. Ensure that you have a recent line manager's reference. If you have any doubt, or if there are missing key details, or any inconsistency, then ring the referees directly to check and ask them, 'If you had a vacancy, would you appoint this individual again?' When asked in such stark terms, people rarely mislead!

As part of the offer of employment, be sure to include a discussion with the preferred candidates of the details of the package, including start date, holiday, training or other conflicting commitments, and confirming terms and conditions. If in any doubt, take advice from your human resources colleagues.

Staff appraisal, development and training

Although a relatively recent feature within the NHS, most organizations now have an appraisal system in place, and information about this will be available through your human resources (or personnel) department. Nevertheless, it is still common to meet staff and ask when their last appraisal meeting was, and to hear the answer 'Never'.

In our view, appraisal is one of the most important tasks that the manager can do. This is because it formalizes the structure and expectation of roles within the immediate work group. Such formalization is also important for the line manager because the appraisal process can identify the pressures upon staff members, and so act as a spotlight upon organization problems that apply to many other members of staff. The appraisal process should also identify unmet training or staff development needs, and it may also highlight any gaps between existing available training and that which is required. In addition the process can bring into focus previously unrecognized interpersonal tensions. Appraisal can also allow the manager and appraisee to refocus the tasks for the coming year, setting new targets or objectives.

The appraiser role can be a difficult one, and requires specific training. It implies having an up-to-date job description, setting periodic and measurable performance targets and being able to address contextual issues. This includes giving feedback (which may or may not be welcome) to managers on how well they are managing. Also the value of appraisal should accumulate over time, in that this year's training targets can build upon courses or training done in the previous year, and be an important source of planning for the career development for individual staff. The following list (based on Randell, in Sissons 1994) summarizes some of the key functions of the appraisal process:

- evaluation
- auditing
- succession planning
- training
- controlling
- development
- motivation
- validation.

The flexible and understanding employer

While the material terms and conditions that most NHS employees are offered are usually tightly constrained, shrewd managers will keep abreast of the important issues for local staff and will try to minimize their adverse effects by offering staff a range of additional benefits or forms of recognition. Many of these will have a limited financial impact but they can have huge value for staff who feel they are genuinely listened to, and whose difficulties are reflected in specific responses. These benefits will need to address the actual sources of dissatisfaction of staff, not the managers' assumptions about these. Considerable research has been carried out on the factors affecting staff's experience of work. According to Warr (1987), the main categories are:

- opportunities for control
- opportunities for skill use
- externally generated goals
- variety
- environmental clarity
- availability of money
- physical security
- opportunity for interpersonal contact
- valued social position.

The types of responses which may begin to address some of the themes listed include: improvements in the working environment (e.g. iced water machines, fans and blinds for hot weather), basic equipment (e.g. pagers and mobile phones, foot or wrist rests for computers), improved facilities (access to key books or journals, or attractive staff rest rooms and furniture).

The manager can also offer flexibility in terms of the way staff work. For example, at the organizational level, job-sharing, flexitime, sabbaticals, career breaks, part-time contracts and pre-retirement support may need to be introduced, both as good practice but also just to recruit up to complement, and to retain valuable staff. These new options reflect wider changes in social structure characterized, for example, by increasing numbers of women in the NHS who are the primary bread-winners for their families, or by staff who may need to change their contribution to the workplace at different times during their career to take account of varying family responsibilities. Other issues may cause significant frustration or demoralization for staff and cannot be resolved at your local level, and will be need to be passed on to senior managers for an organization-wide response, for example the provision of nursery, child care and holiday playschemes, access to proper parking, or support for affordable housing, especially for lower-paid staff.

Helping those who struggle

In any work group there will be staff who struggle. We propose a four-step approach to address this problem: (i) identify, (ii) diagnose, (iii) structure, and (iv) formalize. The *identification* must come first, before you will be able to deal with these problems. This can be achieved by the direct report of staff who are not performing well. Indirect reports from colleagues are also common, although they may be 'anonymized' and should be verified to avoid scapegoating. Complaints from users, carers or other agencies may highlight such problems. Failure to meet project or appraisal targets can be important, also poor attendance or sickness records. In addition, you will need to be keen in your observations of which staff often appear tired, irritable, uncooperative, anxious or poorly organized, all of which can be indicators of incipient or already developed difficulties.

Having identified staff with possible problems, how can you *diagnose* the underlying issues? In terms of the context, such difficulties can arise for many reasons. Mental health services continue to change rapidly, and so previous training may be less and less relevant today. Individuals might have been moved unwisely into their current posts, or been restructured around, or inappropriately promoted. These kinds of problems affecting staff members usually fall into the following categories:

- their job is poorly defined
- the volume of their work is not achievable
- their responsibilities are too great
- they need training (including knowledge updating)
- they have never been clearly managed before
- they have burnout or poor motivation
- they have personal problems (health, alcohol, drugs, debt, family)
- they are in a job not suited to them.

The third step is to offer a *structured approach* to performance management. This means meeting with the person concerned (do not tackle these problems by mail!), saying that you have identified a problem, offering your diagnosis or interpretation, and listening to their response. Commonly the staff member will reveal a series of background difficulties that make their current poor performance more understandable. Even so you will need to proceed to negotiate a series of clear, achievable, timetabled and realistic objectives aiming to improve and monitor work performace. This may also include offering training, counselling, mentoring, secondments, or agreed periods of compassionate, study or special leave. This process must be documented, both for the manager and for the employee, and should form part of a regular review procedure. With this type of structure and support most staff improve in their performance. When they do not, then you may need to *formalize* the process, by closely following your organization's staff performance and disciplinary procedures. These may include the options of disciplinary actions, redeployment, medical or early retirement, or, in extreme cases, redundancy.

Good practice in supervision

Staff working in mental health services often feel high levels of stress for several reasons. Their work sets unusual demands. Staff will have to deal with service users whose behaviour may be odd or bizarre, and occasionally may be disturbed, or disturbing. Sometimes service users are verbally or physically aggressive or threaten suicide. For all these reasons clinical and managerial staff need to be continually vigilant and to be prepared for attacks upon their physical or psychological integrity.

There is also a current trend for the community and some parts of the media to blame staff for the symptoms and behaviours indicative of mental illness among the service users they treat and do their utmost to assist. In response to these pressures, a clear structure of regular clinical supervision is vital for all staff. In our experience mental health teams often allow clinical supervision to cease as a result of the pressures they are under. We would argue that clinical supervision structures are essential to underpin effective team working, and become more important at times of stress, change and instability. There are several useful models of supervision available, or a team can agree their own structure and process locally. The general principles of supervision should include:

- an expectation that supervision is the norm and not the exception for the service and staff
- an agreed contract between supervisor and supervisee (including frequency, duration, content, confidentiality and location of supervision)
- clarification of the responsibility of the supervisor to arrange, facilitate and provide alternatives if supervisor not available
- agreement on who and what is being noted as part of supervision
- agreement on whether supervision will be individual or with a group of peers
- appropriate training and supervision for supervisors themselves.

In this section we have deliberately emphasized the importance of supervision, which could be seen as analogous to regular car maintenance. For both, if routinely conducted, problems can be identified early and resolved efficiently. If either are not done, or not done well, minor difficulties become major problems that can lead to underperformance or complete breakdown. An alternative image to underscore the central organizational importance of supervision is to see it as a cascade of supplies, or as nourishment which flows throughout the organization. In this metaphor we can see that if supervision is not supplied to a middle manager, then they will not be sustained to provide sufficient flow of supervision to those below them in the hierarchy. This can be seen as a form of organizational anorexia or malnutrition that is avoidable or indeed reversible once it has been identified and its importance appreciated.

Preventing burnout

A limited amount of stress is necessary to increase work performance. Handy (1976) has distinguished the beneficial role of stress (role pressure) from the harmful role of stress (role strain). He pointed out that one of the major tasks of management is to control the level of stress in organizations. The symptoms of role strain are tension, low morale and communication difficulties.

The term *burnout* has come to be widely used and recognized as the consequence of prolonged and severe role strain. Burnout has been defined by Maslach and Jackson (1979) as a dysfunctional psychological state that occurs especially in conditions with high levels of personal interaction, along with chronic stress and tension. These conditions are frequently found in community mental health teams, which we consider to be continually at risk of staff burnout. The characteristics and causes of burnout have been summarized by Mosher and Burti (1994):

Description
1 no energy
2 no interest in service users
3 service users seen as frustrating, hopeless or untreatable
4 higher absenteeism
5 high staff turnover
6 demoralization.

Causes
1 setting too hierarchical: staff not empowered
2 too many externally introduced rules, no local authority and responsibility
3 work group too large or non-cohesive
4 too many service users: staff feel overwhelmed
5 too little stimulation, too much routinization.

To deal with role strain, Handy (1976) has identified the following strategies: repression, withdrawal and rationalization. In *repression* the individual refuses to admit that there is any problem. In *withdrawal* the individual retreats behind a psychological barrier or leaves the organization. In *rationalization* the individual decides that the conflict is inevitable and must be lived with. Managers will therefore need to be ready to identify these symptoms, preferably at an early stage. Once identified, the manager will need to work with the member of staff to acknowledge the problem, to try to understand the particular issues that combine to exert the pressure experienced by that individual. The vital next step, however, is to offer a structured plan to reverse the level of burnout; the principles that apply here are those we outlined above in the section where we discussed staff who struggle.

Community mental health teams also offer staff positive work experiences, which can mitigate against burnout. Staff are likely to have different types of opportunities for control. Relatively junior staff are also often allowed greater degrees of clinical discretion in their treatment plan for service users, within a context of supervision and professional support, than is usually the case in hospital settings. The wide variety of clinical problems presenting to a community mental health team will provide many opportunities for skill use, when members of different disciplines can exercise their specific professional skills.

Variety is additionally important in avoiding burnout. In many clinical teams increased variety may be a positive aspect of community services that include visits to service users' homes, or to other non-institutional sites. A further important contextual feature of workplaces that aim to minimize burnout is clarity within the organizational environment. This requires the work setting to be clear in three senses: the availability of feedback on the consequences of one's actions, the degree to which the actions of other people are predictable, and the clarity of role expectations.

Conclusion

In this chapter we have put forward one central idea: that mental health services are no more than the sum of the skills and commitment of their staff. We see staff as a renewable and scarce resource, which requires a strategy for structured long-term investment. We believe that most staff try their best, and can do better if well managed. There are four key aspects to this developmental approach. (i) As a manager, identify poor performance early and often! (ii) Recruit people to fit the gaps within teams. (iii) Create a structure of regular, predictable and valued supervision and career development. (iv) Establish a clear overall strategic framework within which individual roles make sense.

References and further reading

Frank, J. (1961) *Persuasion and Healing*. New York: Academic Press.

Handy, C. (1976) *Understanding Organisations*. London: Penguin.

Maslach, C. and Jackson, S. (1979) Burned-out cops and their families, *Psychology Today*, 12: 59–62.

Mosher, L. and Burti, L. (1994) *Community Mental Health. Principles and Practice*, 2nd edn. New York: Norton.

Prosser, D., Johnson, S., Kuipers, E., Szmukler, G., Bebbington, P. and Thornicroft, G. (1996) Mental health, 'burnout', and job satisfaction among hospital and community-based mental health staff, *British Journal of Psychiatry*, 169: 334–7.

Randell, G. (1994) Employee appraisal, *Personnel Management*, 2nd edn. Oxford: Blackwell.

Roth, A. and Fonagy, P. (1996) *What Works, for Whom? A Critical Review of Psychotherapy Research*. New York: Guildford Press.

Sisson, K. (1994) *Personnel Management*, 2nd edn. Oxford: Blackwell.

Warr, P. (1987) *Work, Unemployment and Mental Health*. Oxford: Oxford University Press.

Watts, F. and Bennett, D. (1983) Management of the staff team, in F.N. Watts and D. Bennett (eds) *Theory and Practice of Psychiatric Rehabilitation*, 313–28. Chichester: John Wiley and Sons.

Task 3 **Managing budgets**

Key themes

In this chapter we aim to:

- give an overview of budgeting in the NHS
- unravel the jargon
- explain who's who in the finance department
- demystify budget statements – giving real examples!
- explain how to implement simple local financial controls
- clarify issues about overspending and underspending.

Accounting, like taxes, has been a function of organised society throughout history. It is the recording, reporting and sometimes interpretation of all the financial (money value) transactions and resources of business enterprises and other formal organizations.

(Glynn *et al.*, *Accounting for Managers* 1994: 1)

Introduction

If you are a manager of staff within the NHS it is likely that you will have the task of managing a *delegated budget*. (Words in italics are defined in the Jargon box on p. 129.) This prospect fills many first-time managers with some level of fear and concern. In this chapter we outline a framework for managing NHS budgets, identify some of the rules about budget management, and take the reader step by step through a budget illustration.

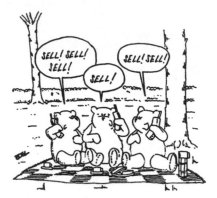

Teddy Bears' Panic

Since the creation of NHS Trusts and GP fundholders after the NHS and Community Care Act 1990, financial responsibility and accountability have been devolved down to *purchaser* and *provider* organizations. Hospital Trusts (as providers) are responsible for managing their allocated annual budgets (both revenue and capital). An NHS accounting year runs from 1 April to 31 March. All monies are allocated for one financial year, and should be spent within each year.

As well as an *annual revenue budget*, which is primarily an agreed contract for services with a purchasing health authority, a Trust may receive a capital allocation. This capital can be 'borrowed' from the Treasury at the agreed public sector borrowing rate and paid back over an agreed period (i.e. a mortgage repayment with interest). The amount a Trust can borrow is stipulated in their *external financing limit* (rather like the maximum mortgage given against a salary). Capital can also be provided as part of a *private finance business case* agreed with the NHS Executive or as a one-off capital allocation (e.g. Tomlinson grants in Inner London). Capital would be required to purchase new buildings, refurbish existing ones or purchase large equipment. In spending an allocated revenue budget there are some basis rules that should be followed by all provider units. These are (according to Glynn and Perkins 1995):

- The price of patient treatment is to be considered as the *full cost* – that is, including an allowance for associated capital costs, such as buildings and equipment, which are no longer to be treated as a 'free good'.
- Purchasers and providers have to achieve *balanced budgets* year on year.
- All levels of management must demonstrate that funds are prudently allocated, expenditure strictly controlled and performance critically examined.

These three simple principles are always reinforced at a local Trust level by written *standing financial instructions*. These are the detailed procedures set out by the director of finance, to which all budget holders must work. These are usually available directly from the office of the director of

Table 11.1   The contracting timetable

Stage	Time
Price procedures	May
Value-for-money market comparisons	June/July
Preliminary purchasing plan	October
Service specification from purchaser	October
Consultation meetings	December/January
Contract negotiations	December/January/February
Firm purchasing plans	November/December
Formal proposals received	January
Negotiations concluded	March
Contracts signed	31 March

Source: Hodgeson and Holie (1996).

Table 11.2   Standard cost classifications

Description	Classification	Analysis
Consultant psychiatrist	fixed	direct
Senior registrar	semi-fixed	direct
Finance director	fixed	overhead
Drugs	variable	usually indirect
Dressings	variable	usually indirect

Source: Glynn and Perkins (1995).

finance. As stated earlier, revenue budgets are negotiated annually between purchasers and providers, and this negotiation occurs within a fixed *contract cycle*. The cycle is described in Table 11.1.

When an NHS provider is negotiating its contract with a particular health authority, the provider must cost in detail all services to be provided. The costs must also be categorized as *fixed*, *semi-fixed* or *variable*. These are important distinctions because the cost of services can fluctuate if the costs are not fixed and controlled, and the purchaser will need to consider this when negotiating a contract. This process is described in more detail in Table 11.2.

While most operational managers will be concerned with the implications of the service contract negotiated between their Trust and the health authority (as this will determine the funding available for the following financial year). The NHS does use other types of contract in its day-to-day work. Some of these are listed in Table 11.3.

Financial language has entered the NHS at a significant rate. Much of it is baffling to clinicians and new managers. The Jargon box outlines some of the most common terms.

Table 11.3   Types of contract in the NHS

Type of contract	Key characteristics
NHS purchaser–provider contract	internal to the NHS and not enforceable in law
Contracts with GPs, dentists, opticians and retail pharmacists	legal contracts with independent businesses negotiated nationally between the government and representative bodies
Contracts of employment	contracts between employers and employees. Governed predominantly by employment law and enforced largely through industrial tribunals
Contracts with non-NHS suppliers	conventional commercial contracts

Source: Hodgeson and Holie (1996).

Who's who in the finance department?

If you are responsible for managing a delegated budget, in addition to understanding the key terms, you will also need to develop a close working relationship with finance department staff. Depending on the size of the department, the first place to start is with either the director or assistant director of finance (responsible for revenue budgets). You will have several questions that you need to ask them when you meet, which will include:

- What are the standing financial instructions for the Trust?
- What budget do they think you manage and can you have details of them?
- What are the reporting procedures on budget performance? (e.g. monthly, two-monthly, quarterly)
- Who arranges for your specimen signature to be taken?
- How much are you authorized to order against your budgets for single purchases? (e.g. £250, £1,000)
- Who will be your regular contact in finance to help you manage your budget?
- Does the department provide any financial training for managers?

Case study   Demystifying budget statements

After this rapid introduction to financial arrangements in the NHS, the language that is used, and some of the people who manage finance in your Trust, we turn next to a practical example of how you as a manager can use your understanding to manage effectively the budgets that have been delegated to you. If you manage a *revenue* budget, you will be given an annual budget statement that will outline (i) the amount of money allocated to your cost centre, and (ii) how it is categorized into budget lines (in other words, areas of expenditure).

Jargon box

annual revenue budget allocated funds for one financial year for a specific *cost centre*

balanced budgets actual spending is no more and no less than allocated budget

capital all costs associated with equipment and building purchases, all of which will be recorded as organizational assets

contract cycle the stages of negotiating, agreeing and signing contracts (see Table 11.2)

cost centre the code to which parts of the budget are allocated by the finance department, e.g. 'Community Mental Health Team South'

cost line the specific coded line on a budget statement to which specific costs are charged, e.g. travelling costs

delegated budget the agreed sum of money for which a specific named manager is responsible and accountable, within a financial year

direct costs the treatment and staff costs of delivering a service, including (for example) secretaries, CPNs and drug budget

end of year the process in the finance department of organization where all charges and income against the given financial year are reconciled against that year's budget. This process allows the production of end-of-year accounts

external financing limit the maximum level of borrowing to raise capital that a Trust is allowed by the NHS Executive

full cost the cost of providing a service that includes *direct*, indirect, *on-costs* and *overheads*

on-costs the costs to the organization of employing a member of staff, including, e.g. National Insurance and pension contributions

overheads the organization's costs of supporting the delivering of a service, a proportion of which is added to direct costs in contracts, e.g. cost of human resources department

private finance business case the formal process by which public sector organizations seek Treasury approval to proceed with a private sector financier in the provision of a public service or building

projected costs the amount the finance department expects to be spent in the future based on past spending patterns

provider an organization contracted to deliver direct NHS services

purchaser an organization buying NHS services on behalf of the NHS Executive, i.e. health authorities

revenue annual allocated funds for the day-to-day running of the service

standing financial instructions written procedures provided by the Trust's director of finance, with which all budget managers must comply

virement the process by which a sum of money allocated to one cost centre is transferred to another

If, for example, you are a ward or service manager for a 12-bed acute in-patient ward, your budget statement for this financial year may look like Table 11.4.

Table 11.4   Annual budget: Patricia ward

Grade	w.t.e.*	w.t.e. e.d.a.†	Basic rate	Max. e.d.a.	Supp.	Total net‡	Budget cost
A	B		C			D	E
Nurse H	1.00	0.00	21,800	0	700	22,500	22,500
	1.00						*22,500*
Nurse F	1.00	0.00	16,500	1,500	700	18,700	18,700
F	1.00	0.00	16,500	1,500	700	18,700	18,700
	2.00						*37,400*
Nurse E	1.00	0.09	14,800	1,200	700	16,700	16,700
E	1.00	0.09	14,800	1,200	700	16,700	16,700
E	1.00	0.09	14,800	1,200	700	16,700	16,700
E	1.00	0.09	14,800	1,200	700	16,700	16,700
E	1.00	0.09	14,800	1,200	700	16,700	16,700
E	1.00	0.09	14,800	1,200	700	16,700	16,700
E	1.00	0.18	14,800	3,200	700	18,700	18,700
	7.00						*118,900*
Nurse D	1.00	0.09	13,200	1,200	700	15,100	15,100
	1.00						*15,100*
Nurse A	1.00	0.09	9,500	500	700	10,700	10,700
A	1.00	0.09	9,500	500	700	10,700	10,700
A	1.00	0.09	9,500	500	700	10,700	10,700
A	1.00	0.09	9,500	500	700	10,700	10,700
A	1.00	0.09	9,500	500	700	10,700	10,700
	5.00						*53,500*
Cost of staffing							247,400
Non-pay							14,000
Total cost							261,400

* whole-time equivalent
† extra duty allowance, paid to nurses for working nights and weekends
‡ total net cost for organization of employee, i.e. salary, London weighting e.d.a., tax, pension

Looking at the annual budget statement for Patricia ward shown in Table 11.4, there are several important characteristics to notice. Column A lists nurses employed by nursing grade. Column B relates this to the actual hours each nurse is paid to work. In this scheme 1.00 means full-time. Column C shows the basic rate of pay each nurse can earn in 12 months. Column D shows the total net maximum pay, and this is an important code for nurses who work shifts because it includes the enhanced hourly rates they can be paid for night or weekend duty. Column E shows the total maximum cost of employing each nurse, and this is a combination of the basic rate of pay, enhancements and employers' National Insurance and pension contributions.

Looking across the rows, each italicized row shows the sub-total of costs and numbers of nurses employed at each grade. At the bottom right-hand corner of the table the total staff costs are shown, in this case, £247,400 for the whole financial year. The bottom right corner also shows the non-pay allocation for the ward in this financial year; in this case the amount is £14,000. 'Non-pay' can be used for the following types of cost: dressings, stationery and general supplies for the ward, patient travel costs, and the costs of daily newspapers.

It is important to know how many staff you have funding to employ and at which grades. In this illustration you are funded to employ 16 full-time nurses. As long as you employ 16 or fewer staff, at this grade-mix, your budget will not be overspent! Notice that the last line of grade E pay w.t.e. e.d.a. shows 0.18, which allows for night pay. So if all your E grades worked night duty you would overspend.

How can you decide if your 16 nursing posts are sufficient to provide 24-hour cover for the ward throughout the year? Table 11.5 shows a method to calculate how many staff you will need to employ to provide a given shift-by-shift staffing level. The calculation is based on the availability of nurses over a 12-month period.

Because a ward is open seven days a week and operates a morning shift of 7.30 a.m. to 3.00 p.m. and an evening shift of 3.00 p.m. to 9.00 p.m., there are 14 day shifts to be covered each week. For nurses to work their contracted hours each week they are all available for five shifts. Each year a nurse gets 36 days annual leave (or 36 shifts); the budget also allows ten days (or shifts) mandatory allowance for training, and the same amount to

Table 11.5   Calculating nursing staff required for a 24-hour shift pattern

Day shifts (morning and evening)

day shifts to cover	14×52 weeks = 728 shifts
staff available	$5 \times 52 = 260$ shifts
annual leave to deduct	(36 shifts)
study days to deduct	(10 shifts)
average sickness, 4%	(10 shifts)
shifts available per staff member per year	204 shifts
staff to shift ratio	*728/204 = 3.56 w.t.e.*

Night shifts

night shifts to cover	$7 \times 10 \times 52 = 3,640$ hours
staff available	37.5×52 weeks = 1,950 hours
annual leave to deduct	(270 hours)
study days to deduct	(75 hours)
average sickness, 4%	(75 hours)
staff available per year	1,530 hours per year
staff to shift ratio	*3,640/1,530 = 2.37 w.t.e.*

cover replacement costs if the nurse is sick during the year. (Note that nights are calculated in hours because the shift is longer and that total contracted hours for night staff are worked over a month, not a week. There are seven nights a week to cover, compared to 14 day shifts.)

In managing your 12-bed in-patient acute ward the Professional Nurse Advisor for the Trust informs you that to give safe and therapeutic nursing care on the ward, you need three nurses on an early shift, three on a late, and two at night. So, using the calculation in Table 11.5 you need to employ 3.56 w.t.e. × 3 = 10.68 w.t.e. nurses for days and 2.37 w.t.e. × 2 = 4.74 w.t.e. nurses for nights. This requires you employing 15.42 w.t.e. nurses in total. As you have 16 w.t.e. nurses funded in your budget, you can accommodate this shift pattern within your budgeted staffing.

From this calculation you may feel reassured that you can run your ward and not overspend your budget. Nevertheless, you also need to be aware of the following factors that could adversely affect your ability to stay within budget and staff the ward safely:

- if sickness of staff goes above the calculated 4 per cent
- if you as the ward manager are asked to work 9 till 5 instead of shifts
- if you require extra staffing to manage difficult patients, over the 3 +3 + 2 establishment
- if staff each take more than 10 days training on average per year.

If you were to find from this calculation that you have a budget for fewer nursing posts than you need to staff the ward safely to the required level, or that the grades of nurses are too low, then you will need to have early discussions with your line manager and with the finance department to consider options to reconcile this shortfall.

Conclusion

The new financial framework of delegated budgets means that most managers now need to understand how to manage these responsibilities effectively. This will mean that you will need to learn more about the wider NHS financial context, and then more about your own financial duties and limitations. By taking you through a worked example we have attempted in this chapter to show you some basic elements in interpreting financial statements. When you have mastered the basics of managing budgets then you will be in a position to run your budgets confidently so that they best fit your service goals, and to enjoy this new challenge in doing so.

References and further reading

Glynn, J., Perrin J. and Murphy, M. (1994) *Accounting for Managers*. London: Chapman and Hall.
Glynn, J. and Perkins, A. (1995) *Managing Health Care – Challenges for the 90s*. London: Saunders.

Hodgeson, K. and Holie, R. (1996) *Managing Health Service Contracts*. London: Saunders.
Iles, V. (1997) *Really Managing Health Care*. Buckingham: Open University Press.

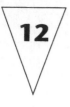

12 / Task 4 Creating a robust infrastructure

> **Key themes**
>
> In this chapter we discuss:
>
> - managing the clinical team
> - how to create a strong infrastructure
> - maintaining a quality service
> - enhancing communication
> - the manager as leader.

In previous chapters we have written as if mental health services must remain in a permanent state of flux. While we know that services have undergone a great deal of change, we believe that these major changes will be relatively rare events. For most of the time, therefore, the main issues facing managers are the consolidation, maintenance and gradual quality improvement of the service elements for which they are responsible. In this chapter we discuss the ways in which mental health service managers can stabilize and maintain their services by providing a robust infrastructure. In considering 'infrastructure' we shall look in turn at: (i) the clinical team and its management, (ii) the quality of the service, (iii) the administration of the service, and (iv) communication. In the final section we shall look at the manager as a leader.

Managing the clinical infrastructure

While the individual staff member is of central importance in providing good quality direct treatment and support to service users, it is the quality of the team that makes the difference between good and bad mental health services. We see the staff team both as made up of individual clinicians, and as an important entity in its own right. The characteristics of a team as a whole are not simply the sum of the parts; they include the clinical setting, the style of leadership, and the degree of coordination with other staff. It is therefore necessary to consider the clinical team as an agent or a vehicle of service provision, separate from the contribution of the individual clinicians.

It can be helpful to think of the team in four stages: *new team building, major reconstruction, maintenance* and *minor reconstruction*. In most cases, what happens is that a new team leader inherits an existing staff group, so the primary questions are how far and how fast to change. Figure 12.1 shows the cyclical relationship between the phases of team maintenance, and initial construction or subsequent reconstruction.

While Stage 1 (new team building) is relatively uncommon, it occurs more often when the service is experimental, in other words when it is supported by research funds from the outset. In this case it will have clear goals, to be achieved within a limited period of time, which are defined by the research purpose. In routine settings, by comparison, there may be limited opportunities to establish completely new services.

At the beginning of a new clinical team, there is the opportunity for the team leaders to influence powerfully the shape and style of the nascent service. Many of the routines and traditions that quickly become institutionalized within work groups are initially absent and can be invented. The allocation of room space, for example, can alter patterns of behaviour in the team, and can also set the tone for more or less hierarchical social relationships between team members. Siting all members of one team in the same or adjacent offices, with private interview rooms bookable for all staff, may go some way to increase communication within a team.

The name of the team can exert a strong influence upon how it is conceived by its own staff and by external agencies. Geographically recognizable names may strengthen the identification of the function of the team by

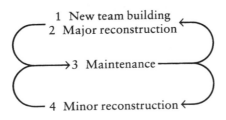

1 New team building
2 Major reconstruction
3 Maintenance
4 Minor reconstruction

Figure 12.1 Cycles of clinical team building, maintenance and reconstruction

outside agencies, but Trusts and also locality teams are now subject to periodic mergers and de-mergers, which can change their relationships with
local catchment areas. Our own preference is for memorable acronyms for
teams, but this is a matter of taste!

The extent to which the goals of the team are explicitly stated, and jointly
developed, by the team may directly impinge upon the team's effectiveness.
Such goals are most often formulated at the stages of initiation or major
reconstruction of a team. Their importance increases when a service under-
goes a period of most intense pressure, such as during a time of rapid staff
turnover, exceptional clinical demand, or staff absence, or in times of external threat, for example of financial cut-backs. At these times a clear statement of the core functions of the team, especially if this has been agreed with
the service commissioners, may be invaluable to use as a point of reference
when reprioritizing, and to provide staff with focus and direction.

Major reconstruction is Stage 2, which in many ways is parallel to that of
establishing a new team. Major reconstruction can occur proactively or
reactively. The first case is usually associated with the arrival of a new team
leader, and this may occur at the service, as well as at the national level,
especially following the election of a new government. The second case,
reactive major construction, is most often found after a perceived system
failure.

At the local level, substantial alterations to mental health teams can
occur in response to changes in clinical leadership, changes in the local
political complexion, from reactions to scandals, or from substantial staff
vacancies. This stage differs from the establishment of a new team, in that
existing staff need to be accommodated within the new structure. Current
service patterns, traditions and customs may prove resistant to alteration,
and there may already be an established set of expectations by service users
and by outside agencies of what services have been offered in the past and
what should be provided in future. Such expectations of staff may be
expressed as a statement of organizational philosophy, for example:

As providers of care and treatment we believe that:
1 Service users are entitled to be offered continuing care, treatment
  and support to enhance their quality of life.
2 Service users are entitled to services which are usually close to home.
3 Service users are entitled to dignity and respect.
4 A one-to-one relationship is a vital component of the service we
  offer.
5 People with mental health problems are entitled to the maximum
  opportunity to develop their potential.
6 Service users are entitled to exercise choice, have control over their
  lives and make contributions appropriate to their abilities and aspir-
  ations.

Stage 3, maintenance, is the most common and probably the most
important of the four stages, as it occupies by far the longest time periods in

the life of a team. It is the most difficult phase as it is routine, but it should not be repetitive. When these maintenance functions are well performed, they are almost invisible. This is exactly the paradox, since there is an absence of positive feedback about good team management, while negative feedback is instantaneous! During the maintenance stage, prior changes to the clinical team will need to be reinforced, for example through initial consultation with staff on the options for change, and at a later stage by regular discussion of how the changes are working in practice, such as at staff away days.

The second essential element in the maintenance stage is setting the boundary conditions. Setting the boundaries of the team work consists of identifying (i) the specific goals and aims of the service in relation to the aims of other local services and agencies, (ii) the particular service user group or groups to be served, for example on the basis of diagnosis or disability, (iii) the intended duration of clinical contact, or of episodes of care, which are indicated by clinical considerations and financial constraints, (iv) the limits of staff tolerance and duty, and (v) the degree to which each particular service acts as a substitute for other service components or for other social support networks, which may be limited, dysfunctional or wholly absent.

These boundaries are entirely necessary for the integrity and sustainability of the work of the clinical team. They may be implicit or explicit, and this is immaterial as long as the team functions effectively. When, however, the team enters a period of relatively poor functioning, then the absence of explicit and written boundaries becomes crucial, as the boundary conditions are not immediately available for review. Without such clear and agreed boundaries, the roles expected of such teams can vary rapidly, and can cause staff anxiety that in itself encourages destabilization and stress.

This is especially the case for teams providing general mental health services for adults, as other specialist or sub-specialist teams can, through effective boundary setting, retreat from whole categories of service users, and the 'general adult' teams are left to act as the default, to treat all those not receiving services from other teams. Unless regulated, this will leave general adult mental health teams feeling that they must take on any service user referred to them, that they have no control over accepting new service users, or over their caseloads, and that they are always either actually, or in danger of being, overwhelmed by their clinical commitments.

The advantage of having clear and realistic boundaries, stating both what the service is able, and is not able, to provide, is that it helps to limit inappropriate demand, and it avoids the additional stress on staff of having to narrow the role of the team at a later stage, with the consequent disappointment of staff and of outside referral agencies. It also gives clear expectations for all staff, and this is especially important when working with people who are severely disabled by mental illness.

Example

We planned to establish a multi-disciplinary community mental health team (CMHT) for a defined geographical sector in South London. No new resources were available for the service, so all the staff for the team were redeployed from other parts of the service, including a day hospital, a CPN team, a local time-limited case management team and an acute in-patient unit. For local reasons (the day hospital was closing) we needed to establish the team quickly, but the structure, boundaries and operational policies for the new CMHT were not yet fully developed, and had not been through a full consultation process. We therefore decided to call the first version of the new team the 'Interim Community Team' so that it was clear to every-one that this was a temporary, transitional, time-limited stage, pending the agreement on the new fully established team, which started one year later.

Stage 4 is that of minor reconstruction, the episodes during which less vital 'running repairs' are conducted to improve a team's effectiveness. This stage is necessary at regular intervals in each service, to monitor the team's performance in relation to changing conditions and because a moderate degree of change is important for staff morale. This also depends upon the ability of the team to diagnose dysfunction in their own work at an early stage, before the point at which major reconstruction becomes necessary.

Common occasions for minor reconstruction are times of limited staff turnover. Such changes can also occur in reaction to the injection of ideas from visitors to the team, from visits of staff to teams elsewhere; they can arise from an appreciation of the research literature, from relatively minor budgetary changes, or from external 'diagnosticians' who may be group facilitators who are brought in temporarily to suggest minor improvements or small-scale changes. Whatever the source of the ideas, the phase of minor reconstruction is important to fix problems early, and as an antidote to the routinization of everyday work. At a time of minor reconstruction it is useful to check for evidence of staff burnout or (at the opposite end of the scale) staff satisfaction from their experience in the team.

Within the clinical team, there are a number of techniques to prevent and reverse burnout, including didactic training exercises, regular staff meet-ings for interpersonal problem resolution, routine case conferences to dis-cuss difficult cases, and regular supervision (Mosher and Burti 1994). In addition there are a number of features of community mental health teams which encourage functional rather than dysfunctional performance: small team size (usually 6–12), more open patterns of decision making, mutual support and consultation between staff members.

Community mental health teams can also offer additional sources of staff satisfaction. Firstly, the move away from traditional roles and leadership structures may give staff from disciplines such as nursing considerably greater autonomy and responsibility, which may increase their job satis-faction and sense of mastery. Secondly, service users and relatives appear often to prefer community-based care to hospital care, and staff may feel happier about their work when the recipients are more satisfied. Thirdly, staff may feel that their work is more effective when they move into the community. Finally, the traditional psychiatric hospital may be experienced by staff as well as service users as a depressing and institutionalizing environment, and community mental health centres, primary care health centres and service users' homes may in general be more pleasant and stimulating work settings (Prosser *et al.* 1996).

Managing the quality infrastructure

In health care settings the word 'quality' is frequently used, but it is not often understood in detail by staff. Many references to it are made by the government in a continued drive for a 'quality service'. Yet what does the jargon really mean for a mental health service? And how can a manager develop and measure it?

According to Fitzsimmons and Fitzsimmons (1994), service quality has five dimensions:

1 reliability
2 responsiveness
3 assurance
4 empathy
5 tangibles.

The precise quality measures used locally will include some features agreed with outside agencies and some internal to the team or service. Some examples of quality indicators are outlined in Table 12.1.

While all the measures outlined in Table 12.1 impact on the team, some will be national or organizational policy targets, while others will be agreed locally. For a service to be effective the manager needs to be clear about the quality targets placed upon the organization by national policy, ways to communicate their relevance to team members, and how to develop systems to ensure that they are measured. It is important for the clinical team to be involved in discussions about quality of care and about which quality indicators to adopt locally. This may be done annually as part of a team review structure, or through team business meetings.

Managing the administrative infrastructure

As the manager for a given part of a mental health organization, you will be expected to establish a framework of efficient administration for staff whom you manage. This will include the provision of trained secretarial support for staff, the timely circulation of rotas and working procedures (for example, for sickness reporting and for forward planning of annual leave), and overseeing the management of clinical caseloads. In addition, you will need to make the most efficient use of the resources available to

Table 12.1   Indicators of mental health service quality

Dimension	Measure	Level
1 Reliability	• complaints	organization
	• service user satisfaction survey	organization and team
2 Responsiveness	• all referrals seen within two weeks	organization
	• all crises attended to within 24 hours	team
3 Assurance	• reduction in suicides among mentally ill	national
	• prompt investigation of all serious incidents	organization
	• public inquiry into homicides	national
4 Empathy	• involvement of service users in service development	local
	• consultation with black and ethnic minority community	organization
5 Tangible	• minimum staffing levels on in-patient wards	organization or local

you, and to create and maintain the boundary conditions described earlier in this chapter. A well-administered service will need to agree mandatory training for all staff and professional ongoing training, along with training that supports team development. It is important for the manager to compile a record of the targets and individual training profiles and to keep them on file.

We shall illustrate here the particular importance of creating and maintaining boundary conditions with reference to bed management strategies, and to identify ways to define which service users should be targeted by an adult mental health service. As a team manager you may have responsibility for an in-patient service. You will then need to consider a number of bed management strategies, some of which have been described by Strathdee *et al.* (1996). The following list offers a framework for bed management. For any strategy to be effective we suggest that the following list is used as a guide to generate local discussion and a local protocol, with input from many groups of staff, particularly those who work extended hours or night duty.

- *Organization of service*: the sectorization of psychiatric services allows the organization of psychiatric services for the whole population.
- *Site of assessment*: initial assessment should be undertaken at home. Where assessments take place at the site of the acute beds, the likelihood of inappropriate admission is increased.
- *Senior gate-keeping*: where senior doctors or nurses are constantly involved in any decision to admit a service user, their ability to make a

more informed decision and to take risks more appropriately decreases hospital admissions.

- *Bed manager*: in services where an experienced nurse provides a triage function, bed use is likely to be decreased.
- *Discharge planning*: in the event of a homeless person being admitted, if priority is placed on immediate referral to housing services, inappropriate and extended use of beds can be prevented.
- *Continuity of care*: the most likely time of readmission and suicide attempts is in the first four to six weeks after discharge. Out-patient appointments may be appropriately given within this timescale rather than at a later stage. Any follow-up by key workers, case managers, care managers, CPNs or others is more likely to be successful if it is intense in this vulnerable period.
- *Urgent out-patient services*: where urgent out-patient appointments can be offered as part of a comprehensive service, this reduces the need for in-patient admissions.
- *Integrated hospital and community services*: research has demonstrated that without an integrated approach where community teams have control over their own hospital beds, both bed use and length of stay are significantly increased and continuity of care is decreased.

In terms of targeting and prioritizing services it is useful to start with an understanding of the scope of the problem. In any year, up to a quarter of the adult population will suffer from some mental health problem that interferes with their everyday life. Mental health services in England, however, have the capacity to treat only about 1 per cent of the whole population at any one time. The continuing question for mental health services is therefore *which 1 per cent?*

Over the last decade national mental health policy has made it clear that services should first serve those who are most disabled by mental illnesses. As yet there is no consensus on how to define this group, which is usually called the 'severely mentally ill' (SMI). In many local areas a working definition of the SMI is reached pragmatically – often based on agreed priorities for local rehabilitation services – for service users to be included in the Care Programme Approach (CPA), or to receive care management services. As a manager, one of the central operational tasks you may face in working with the clinical team is to agree how to decide (i) which referred service users to assess, (ii) which assessed service users to take on for an episode of treatment, and (iii) reasonable grounds for discharging service users back to the primary care services. Some of the most useful practical definitions of SMI are given in Table 12.2.

Managing the communication infrastructure

One of the most frequently heard complaints of clinical and managerial staff in health services is that they do not receive sufficient communication

Table 12.2   Definitions of the severely mentally ill

Goldman (1981)
Diagnosis: service users diagnosed according to DSM-III-R criteria with these three conditions:
- schizophrenia and schizo-effective drug (ICD9 295)
- bipolar disorders and major depression (ICD9 296)
- delusional (paranoid) disorder (ICD9 297).

Duration: at least one year since onset of disorder
Disability: sufficient to impair seriously role performance in at least one of the following areas:
- occupation
- family responsibilities
- accommodation.

McLean and Liebowitz (1989)
At least one of the following must be present:
1 two or more years' contact with services
2 depot prescribed
3 ICD9 295 or 297
4 three or more in-patient admissions in the last two years
5 three or more day-patient episodes in the last two years
6 DSM-III-R highest level or adaptive functioning in the past year, level 5 or less.

Tyrer *et al.* (1993)
- service users with chronic psychosis
- two or more in-patient admissions in the past year
- contact with two/more psychiatric agencies in the past year
- frequent consultations
- risk of being imprisoned.

Audit Commission (1994), derived from Patmore and Weaver (1991)
- psychotic diagnosis, organic illness or injury *and* previous compulsory admission *or* aggregate one-year stay in hospital in the past five years *or* three or more admissions in the past five years
- psychotic diagnosis, organic illness or injury *or* any previous admissions in the past five years
- no record of hospital admissions *and* no recorded psychotic diagnosis, organic illness or injury.

---

on matters that affect them. It is therefore important for the team manager to devise and implement a communication plan. As stated in previous chapters, any communication should build upon and enhance a pre-existing supervision structure for all staff. The communication plan should therefore outline what other communication channels or forums will be used in the service. Communication planning should not concentrate on communication within the team alone, but also on how to engage service users actively in commenting on local services. For example:

- agree on the principle that you will consult with service users at every possible stage

- identify a well-respected member of staff to coordinate the service user input
- listen to service users' experience of prejudice
- support them in 'practising' to gain confidence in public speaking
- be patient and try to work differently (not everyone enjoys formal meetings!)
- involve service users in making decisions about the local services
- ensure they are asked to join 'real' decision-making groups
- users can be very powerful public relations officers when dealing with the community, but remember it can be painful for users to hear undiluted prejudice
- persevere, as you will need to build the trust of users before they engage with you!

Managers as service leaders

In describing some of the important infrastructure elements of mental health services, we cannot underestimate the importance of the managerial role and the contribution that managers make to create and maintain robust systems. This is pivotal, particularly if a service is clearly struggling. John Øvretveit, in the book *Coordinating Community Care* (1993), has stressed the team leader's importance:

> More team problems are caused by inadequate team leadership than by any other single factor. Problems rarely come about because the leader is inadequate for the work – it is more likely that his or her formal leadership role is not clear.
>
> (Øvretveit 1993)

We have already considered in Chapter 10 the importance of 'getting the right people, in the right jobs', along with the importance of staff having clear job roles and regular supervision. This approach is vital for all staff and is equally important when considering the team leader role. Many problems are likely to remain unresolved throughout the service if the leadership role within the team is not well defined. Some examples of the problems encountered are:

- profession or line managers may over-control their staff, making it difficult for them to contribute to the team
- managers may under-control their staff, because they assume that the team or team leader is doing the necessary management work
- managers are unsure of their accountability for their staff in the team, and the accountability of the team leader
- staff do not know who to go to for a decision
- some team members are tempted to exploit such lack of clarity to get their own way, for example by telling the team that their manager will not allow them to undertake a task, when no one knows whether this is true

- the team leader's authority to uphold a team policy is not clear. He or she may not be able to find out or act if a team member does not follow the policy. This undermines the credibility of the policy and devalues the work everyone has put into creating it
- channels and responsibilities for complaints are unclear: should a person go to the team leader or to a team member's manager, or to someone else?

In conclusion, in this chapter we have described the hybrid responsibilities as necessary for creating and consolidating the service infrastructure, but they are complex. They are in many ways different from the skills required by managers only ten years ago for the successful delivery of services that were mostly sited in psychiatric hospitals. These new types of responsibilities therefore require a reorientation, a wider view that sees 'outside agencies' not as 'outsiders' but as potential partners. We shall go on to discuss this further in Chapter 13.

References and further reading

Fitzsimmons, J.A. and Fitzsimmons, M.J. (1994) *Service Management for Competitive Advantage*. New York: McGraw Hill.

Goldman, H. (1981) Defining and counting the chronically mentally ill, *Hospital and Community Psychiatry*, 32: 21–7.

Hales, C. (1993) *Managing Through Organisation*. London: Routledge.

La Monica, E. (1990) *Management in Healthcare*. London: Macmillan.

McLean, E. and Liebowitz, J. (1989) Towards a working definition of the long-term mentally ill, *Psychiatric Bulletin*, 13: 251–2.

Mosher, L. and Burti, L. (1994) *Community Mental Health. Principles and Practice* (2nd edn). New York: Norton.

Øvretveit, J. (1993) *Coordinating Community Care. Multidisciplinary Teams and Care Management*. Buckingham: Open University Press.

Patmore, C. and Weaver, T. (1991) *Community Mental Health Teams. Lessons for Planners and Managers*. London: Good Practices in Mental Health.

Powell, R. and Slade, M. (1996) Defining severe mental illness, in G. Thornicroft and G. Strathdee (eds) *Commissioning Mental Health Services*. London: HMSO.

Prosser, D., Johnson, S., Kuipers, E., Szmukler, G., Bebbington, P. and Thornicroft, G. (1996) Mental health, 'burnout', and job satisfaction among hospital and community-based mental health staff, *British Journal of Psychiatry*, 169: 334–7.

Strathdee, G., Davies, S., Perry, M. and Thompson, K. (1996) Commissioning and managing hospital and community beds, in G. Thornicroft and G. Strathdee (eds) *Commissioning Mental Health Services*. London: HMSO.

Tyrer, P., Higgs, R. and Strathdee, G. (1993) *Mental Health and Primary Care. A Changing Agenda*. London: Gaskell and The Mental Health Foundation.

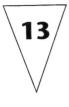

13 | *Task 5* **Allies or adversaries?**

*with Dr Richard Byng and
Sally Pitts-Brown*

Key themes

In this chapter we aim to help you:

- appreciate the mental health service culture shift in the last decade
- understand the key interfaces for adult mental health services
- develop an understanding of the local service context
- identify your key local partners and stakeholders
- open up channels of communication
- establish or join structures that allow collaboration.

Introduction

There has been a remarkable shift of culture within mental health services over the last decade. These changes would make current services almost unrecognizable to a professional who went overseas to work in the mid-1980s and who has now returned to work in the UK. These changes are characterized by:

- a change of the location of services from a few, large institutions to many, decentralized, smaller facilities
- the publication of many more policy requirements and guidelines than ever before
- an explicit expectation that individual professional groups will coordinate with colleagues in multi-disciplinary teams their contributions to service users' treatment and care

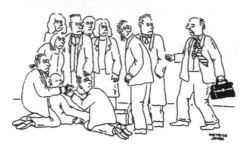

*'Quick, let me through! I'm a Primary Health
Care Provider'*

- firmer policies from central government, requiring that priority is given first to those with the most severe disabilities associated with mental illness
- an increasingly influential role for primary care in the purchasing and commissioning of all health services
- a clearer governmental requirement that NHS services must cooperate with local authority and the independent sector to plan and provide an integrated pattern of local services
- a new attention to the active roles expected of service users and their carers in shaping services
- new governmental guidance to make mental health services more transparent by instigating public inquiries into serious adverse events
- the redirection of mentally ill offenders from the criminal justice system into mental health services, including new court and prison assessment procedures
- a rapidly growing emphasis upon risk assessment and management.

This rapid deluge of complex new policies and procedures has meant that many direct care staff and their managers are only partially informed of the detail, suffer from information overload, and do not always fully appreciate the scale of this massive culture shift.

To help clarify this complicated picture, Figure 13.1 shows a simplified scheme of the whole system, which puts the adult community mental health services in the context of (i) other key NHS services and (ii) other statutory and independent sector providers. The figure shows that there are now many important co-providers. It is important to recognize that a well-functioning mental health network first needs to be constructed from these sometimes fragmented components, and then needs to be developed. This will require managers in particular to have good working relationships with their equivalents in the other corresponding teams, agencies or organizations. This is no simple task! As Figure 13.1 shows, a malfunctioning interface between any two components of the system may reduce the effectiveness of the whole system, and will be likely to have knock-on effects in other parts of the service system. For example, if service users needing high-support residential care cannot move into such provision when needed,

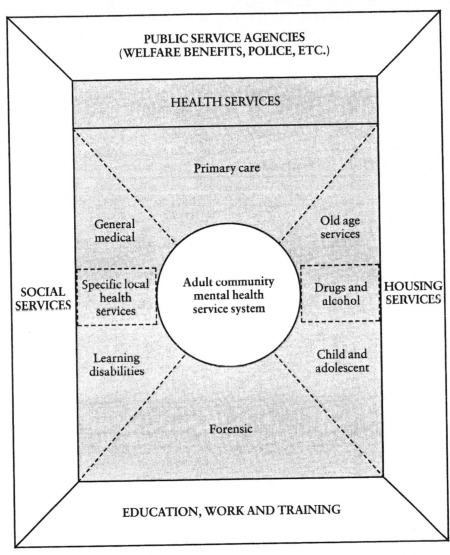

Figure 13.1 Key interfaces between the community mental health service system and (i) other health services and (ii) other public service agencies

they are likely to languish inappropriately on acute psychiatric wards. Similarly, if close joint working is not well established between adult and addiction services, then those service users with both psychotic disorders and substance abuse (often referred to as 'dual diagnosis') will be poorly served.

In this chapter we propose a four-step framework to coordinate these multiple interfaces and relationships:

1 Develop an understanding of the agencies in the local service context, their incentives, drivers, priorities, limitations, and their organizational cultures.
2 Identify your key local partners and stakeholders, and find out details of their natural habitat, including where they work and where they meet.
3 Open up channels of communication.
4 Establish or join structures that allow collaboration across these interfaces and boundaries.

Understanding the local service context

The first step is to develop a detailed understanding of your local scene. This will include making an inventory of all the agencies providing a local service for people with mental health problems. In most situations such a directory will not exist, and this will take a little detective work. Usual sources of information about counselling or self-help or community services, for example, are local libraries or leisure centres. Other key sources will be the local housing department, social services information desks and primary care staff. A further potential goldmine of information is to ask for the advice of staff who have lived and worked in the local area for many years.

In the process of doing this you may want to compile a guide to local services. Commonly such a process will list many organizations who were previously unknown to health services staff and to which cross-referrals can now be made. Such a process implies an important change of orientation for NHS mental health staff, away from a view that they alone provide for people with mental illnesses to a perspective that appreciates that they are a part of one of the many organizations that interact to provide a pattern of care. The key distinction here is between (i) the treatment and care *services* provided by individual agencies, and (ii) the whole mental health care *system*, comprising the separate service components.

It is useful to compile such an inventory when first coming into post (when you can arrange to meet staff at other agencies, and offer or feign complete ignorance of the local scene, as part of your induction). Equally this process can be undertaken at the start of a new planning process, for example when writing or revising the local mental health strategy or the operational policy for one service component. In this case you can describe this work as part of a local 'fresh start'.

During this process you will need to develop a sensitive appreciation of the differing formal responsibilities of the main service provider organizations and their distinct cultural differences. Table 13.1 summarizes some of the formal organizational differences between the four main provider sectors: NHS, social services, voluntary and charitable bodies, and user-led organizations.

To understand better the responsibilities shown in Table 13.1 you will need to keep in mind that there have been three further important trends in

Table 13.1 Overview of the functions of mental health services

Agency	NHS	Social services	Voluntary/charity organizations	Self-help and user-led organizations
Responsibilities	mental and physical health needs (statutory)	social needs (statutory)	social and mental health (non-statutory)	social and mental health (non-statutory)
Who they are	GPs psychiatrists psychologists psychiatric nurses occupational therapists other therapists	social workers care managers home helps home support workers	volunteers and professionals users/carers/local community	former and current service users
What they purchase or provide	CMHT medical treatment psychological treatments in-patient services day hospitals/centres home treatment out-patient services	CMHT residential care supported housing day centres meals on wheels home help benefits advice advocacy	day centres befriending supported housing support groups counselling holidays	self-help advocacy user empowerment education information counselling support groups

Source: Thompson *et al.* (1995).

Table 13.2 Differences in organizational culture between mental health service provider organizations

Organization	NHS	Social services	Voluntary/charities	Self-help and user-led
Accountable to	Secretary of State via NHS Executive	elected councillors and their constituents	to their own board, steering group of funders	Varies: may have formally constituted reporting arrangements or report directly to their members
Planning period	one-year contracts and three- to five-year planning planning cycles for larger projects or local mental health strategies	usually one-year contracts, within the term of office of the elected council	usually determined by the duration of their contracts, or core funding	Often short-term and reliant on limited financial help and on volunteer work and goodwill
Staff training	basic and higher staff training via professional organizations, followed by in-house updates	same as NHS. Non-professional staff usually receive in-house training only	variable. May be linked to statutory sector. Sometimes poorly organized	limited unless linked to national networks of associated organizations
Freedom of speech	subject to professional codes of conduct and NHS policies, including confidentiality	greater formal transparency of communication, with policy/political limitations	greater freedom of speech	greater freedom of speech
Size of organization	very large: Trusts often have 800 to 3,000 staff	very large: social services may have over 500 staff	small: often 30 to 50 staff	very small: often 10 to 20 members in each local group
Funding sources	Department of Health via NHS Executive	Department for Environment and local Council Tax to local authorities	contracts with statutory commissioners, charitable grants, foundations and trustees	limited, some access to statutory grant aid

Table 13.2 (continued)

Organization	NHS	Social services	Voluntary/charities	Self-help and user-led
Funding security	high, annually reviewed	moderate to high, depends on annual central government allocations and local political decisions	low to medium. Varies according to the balance of core and project funding and length of contracts	low. Effectiveness may be limited by continuous funding uncertainties
Statutory and legal responsibilities	many, including the National Health Service Act, Mental Health Act, and the NHS and Community Care Act	many including Children Act, the NHS and Community Care Act, and the Carer Act	several, including regulations that apply to statutory providers if subcontracted	often none
Perceptions of mental illness and treatment	largely medical model: assess, diagnose and treat	usually social model, in family and social context	varies: medical, social or anti-psychiatric model	often anti-medication and for user-involvement at every stage
Focus on individual or family	individual usually	individual within the family context	varies: individual, family or wider community	usually on individual service needs, developing a collective user voice

recent years. First, there is an increasing recent tendency for social services to operate as service brokers rather than as direct service providers, and in particular to buy residential care services and supported housing from the independent sector, for example from housing associations. Second, at the same time there is a shift of some secondary mental health services into primary care. Third, it has become increasingly common for service users and carers and their representative organizations to be directly involved in all stages of planning and commissioning services.

In addition to these time trends, there remain often very significant differences in the organizational culture of the main mental health service providers (Table 13.2). It is very important for managers to understand these differences because if you are going to work closely with people, you need to know where they are coming from! In other words, unless you have a keen appreciation of the constraints and strengths of your potential partner organizations, your dealings with them could be characterized by misunderstanding and frustration.

Identify key local partners and stakeholders

When starting to identify key local partners it may be useful to distinguish between those people who have *formal power* and those with *informal influence*. Those with formal power at the local level are the individuals who occupy the senior positions within their respective organizations. These people are readily identifiable and they will usually include:

Local authority
- director of social services
- director of housing
- director of planning
- local councillors, especially committee chairs.

NHS
- chief executives
- board members
- Community Health Council secretary
- leading GPs
- your equivalent managers in other health Trusts
- senior health authority staff.

Independent and voluntary sector
- directors of housing associations
- directors or heads of charities
- chairs or coordinators of user and carer groups.

By comparison, those with informal influence will often be much harder to identify. These are the people who preside over key organizational crossroads, who have usually been around for at least several years, whose advice is sought by the heads of the statutory organizations, and who will

characteristically have manoeuvred their way onto key financial committees. To succeed with local inter-agency initiatives you must have these
people on your side. To identify them consider using a search pattern technique. On your induction, for example during your visits to formal senior
figures, ask their advice on who else in the local area you should make contact with, and use triangulation: in other words, if one name is mentioned
three or more times, consider contacting that person!

Another similar approach is to identify who is seen locally as having completed a successful project, for example in a parallel organization, such as a
community health or learning disabilities Trust, and when meeting that
person ask who was most practically helpful in realizing their plans. Such
key individuals could, for example, be in the local council planning department, a well-connected church minister, or a residents' association secretary who has a strong local social and political network.

Open up channels of communication

Having established your list of key local figures, you will need to meet them
with the aim of building up good working relationships with them. We suggest that you always offer to arrange your first meeting with that person on
their own territory, or on neutral ground. This is because you will show that
you are making an effort to go more than halfway to meet, to know where
they work, and to add to your understanding of their organizational context. Also, you may well be introduced to other colleagues who are potentially important contacts for collaborative services developments in the
future. Third, a meeting at their site will allow them to give you immediately copies of important documents, such as strategic plans. Fourth, you
are more likely to hear about options for new projects or for calls for bids
for funds at an early stage. Finally, by visiting in this way it may be easier for
your host to give you more detailed information about the recent historical
background to local developments, and this contextual knowledge may be
invaluable to you in the future.

Use structures for collaboration

After meeting these key people in other parts of the mental health service
system, you may be ready to begin on meaningful collaboration. This will
have two aims: to improve current practice and to initiate new service
developments. For both you may need to be highly pragmatic to seize any
opportunity to extend the capacity or the quality of services. First, these
may be in formal organizational settings. Such formal structures, which can
be used for building collaboration, may be standing committees or time-
limited working groups. They usually meet at planned, regular intervals,
have agendas and minutes and an agreed and often representative membership. While they manage the normal capital and revenue streams, and
contain most mainstream initiatives, they usually move slowly, do not

actively encourage creative solutions to local problems, and may meet with insufficient frequency to respond to unexpected short-term funding opportunities, or to rapidly emerging local concerns. Some examples of such formal structures are:

- the chief officer's meeting
- the Joint Planning Team (or Group)
- specific national initiatives (e.g. Health Action Zone)
- Mental Health Act liaison groups
- the hospital reprovision planning team
- primary care groups
- voluntary sector forums and councils
- health and social service integration working groups
- time-limited project groups, e.g. policy for vulnerable adults
- Health Improvement Plan meetings.

In addition, you may wish to take advantage of *informal* opportunities to strengthen your local contacts by joining existing networks or by gathering key individuals together to create a new informal grouping. This can be important when formal structures are ineffective, to be able to respond quickly to short-term funding initiatives, or to develop a coordinated inter-agency approach that can be implemented through the formal structures. For example, the exchanges that occur just before or after formal meetings, or during the breaks at training sessions or conferences, may be more constructive than those that occur in the planned meetings! Such contacts can be invaluable to gather information quickly about what are the hottest current concerns of your colleagues, to sound out views at the earliest possible stage about possible service initiatives, and subsequently to coordinate and strengthen responses to consultation exercises. In our experience, once you have a 'first-name basis' relationship with your equivalents in the other local organizations, you may have the foundation to work in partnership on the larger issues that could never previously be tackled by one agency alone.

To explore these four steps we next look at two case studies that illustrate the pragmatic way our scheme can be applied in practice. The first case study describes the consultation process preceding the opening of a new day centre. The second gives an example of a process intended to improve communication and collaboration between a community mental health team and the local primary health care services.

Case study 1   Neighbour not nimby

The recent experience of developing community mental health facilities has faced a central, unresolved paradox: should neighbours be kept in the dark about local developments or fully informed? Telling neighbours as little and as late as possible is an understandable reaction by staff who may be worried that local opinion may be hostile, uninformed, and could sabotage community care projects. On the other hand, optimists reason that neighbours will find out about new developments on their doorstep sooner or later, and that their anger will be greater if they discover the truth at a late stage. This section describes how mental health staff and local residents in South London have worked together to develop neighbourhood steering groups (NSGs), which act to minimize prejudice against the mentally ill, and to maximize integration within their local communities. This development came in reply to the concerns expressed by local residents, organizations and shopkeepers to the proposals for the new day centre.

During 1993 the local mental health Trust decided to introduce sectorized community mental health services throughout its local catchment area. As one of the most deprived inner city areas in London it received London Implementation Zone funds, which meant that the Trust could buy a property suitable for a day centre. A potentially suitable converted shop in the middle of a local shopping street in a broadly residential area of South London was identified. The selection of the site was guided by the results of a survey of service users who were asked about the type of day care they wanted to be developed. The premises had been previously used as a shop, and the Trust had to apply to the council planning committee for 'change of use' from commercial to health.

The same day that notice was given to neighbours letting them know that a change of use application was coming before the council, the council was deluged by concerned enquiries from neighbours. To ensure that neighbours were given fuller details of the proposal than were available from the council, senior Trust clinical and managerial staff immediately contacted neighbours to put the full facts of the proposal to them. They met with local residents on several occasions in the front rooms of neighbours' houses, in local nursery schools, and in community centres in the neighbourhood. The following list outlines some of the local stakeholders who were identified as needing to be included in the consultation process:

- residents' associations
- school staff, governors and parents
- shopkeepers
- councillors
- local press
- trade associations
- clergy
- police officers
- social services staff
- Members of Parliament.

Neighbours demanded a much broader and longer meeting to discuss the proposals in more detail. A large public meeting was convened at the police station, where many local people made their concerns utterly clear, and where health, social services and police staff jointly presented their plans and proposed safeguards. After three further public meetings, and three appearances before the planning committee (including the helpful mediation of the local ward councillor), staff and neighbours agreed a compromise plan. The agreement was that the centre would open for hours shorter than originally intended, and on Saturday mornings only if the centre had been running smoothly after an initial six-month pilot period.

It was also agreed to set up an NSG to represent a wide range of local interests and advise the management committee of the day centre. The NSG included neighbours, health and social staff, a local police liaison officer, church representatives, members of the local residents' association, and shopkeepers. The key points to consider when setting up an NSG are:

- seek practical success quickly
- enlist support against proposed budget cuts in the health service
- set up a conduit for local neighbours' complaints
- establish advisory powers
- set standards for response to complaints
- include a very wide range of representation
- respond quickly to queries.

The neighbourhood steering group for this project has now been running successfully for over three years. After initially painstakingly establishing a basis of trust with neighbours, staff had to renew this sense of trust with a practical and consistent reply each time a problem was brought to the steering group. There have been no major incidents causing neighbours concern about their safety. Problems arising have been small but important issues, such as the late collection of rubbish by the Trust's portering staff from the pavement, and noise caused while buildings were being converted. The staff have learned some lessons from working with this neighbourhood steering group. They must:

- be proactive
- give out information sheets
- name a key person for contacts
- negotiate on entry criteria to the facility
- be prepared to compromise
- update neighbours on building works
- arrange evening meetings
- slowly build trust
- explode myths about community care
- listen to neighbours' fears.

This collaborative experience demonstrates that treating neighbours openly, as potential partners and as intelligent people with reasonable concerns, is pragmatic, principled, and a proper base for mental health services that are fully integrated within their local communities.

Case study 2 Improving communication between primary care and CMHTs

The primary health care level has always been the main provider of services to most people with mental health problems. Beyond this, however, a detailed understanding of primary care services is now essential for secondary mental health service managers, because recent changes in the law and in health policy have given primary care an ever more important role. This case study will examine some of the recent changes to primary care and the opportunities for collaboration between primary and secondary care.

Primary care and general practice are closely entwined in the UK. A typical general practice is normally a private business run by a partnership of general practitioners who have agreed a contract with the Secretary of State for Health to provide core general medical services. Practice size may vary from 1,500 to 20,000 service users, depending on the number of partners and their workload. Many senior partners still take all management decisions themselves, while other practices have their own managers.

Some general practitioners are used to working in a team with other professionals employed by different organizations; this experience is often positive, but those practitioners either wanting to retain professional barriers or to push collaboration faster than their larger partner organizations may express more negative attitudes as a result. It has been argued that the primary health care team (PHCT) shows few of the characteristics necessary for a team, and often appears as a collection of professionals, who may have different beliefs and allegiances, and who rarely make time to meet and discuss clinical cases or service developments.

This case study shows that it is possible to work together effectively as a clinical team in primary care, and to collaborate extensively with outside organizations, especially if there is willingness on all sides to compromise and air and accept differences.

GPs have enjoyed increasing influence upon secondary services since the NHS and Community Care Act 1990. Fundholding and multifunds have had some impact (although less so) for mental health services, partly due to their geographical sectorization, and because they have not been able to purchase most mental health services. The 1997 White Paper *The New NHS: Modern, Dependable* seeks to strengthen further the wider role of primary care with the formation of primary care groups that will purchase secondary care, monitor GPs, and provide services currently within the remit of community Trusts. Some emerging themes within primary mental health care are:

- more use of cognitive behavioural therapy for service users with depression, anxiety and somatizing
- proactive management of depression with recall systems, guidelines for treatment, and training for its improved recognition
- active case finding and management of those with moderate to heavy alcohol consumption

- prescription of methadone in collaboration with voluntary and statutory agencies
- organized detection of dementia and depression in old age
- health visitors supported to carry out work with families at risk of child-hood mental health problems
- primary health care teams working closely with community mental health teams in shared care arrangements for service users with long-term mental illness.

Current government and health authority policies are actively encouraging primary care and community mental health teams to work together. A number of different models have emerged, for example:

- *separate primary mental health care teams* – funded by primary care and based in the practice, usually with external psychiatrist support
- *practice-based community psychiatric nurse* – provides the main contact point with the Trust, provides interventions and advice, organizes training, acts as key worker to a majority of cases
- *linked liaison workers* – community mental health workers from the CMHT have limited responsibilities, primarily acting to give advice and act as a communication channel for the practice (not taking on practice cases)
- *hybrid model* – community mental health workers work as part of the community team and provide advice to a linked practice, but they increasingly take on cases from the practice, as agreed by the team manager
- *shifted out-patient model* – the psychiatrist conducts an out-patient clinic in the GP's surgery mostly in the absence of the GP
- *consultation-liaison model* – the psychiatrist attends a primary care meeting to discuss management of service users, after which the psychiatrist sees service users often with the GP.

One example of collaboration across the primary–secondary care interface is the Mental Health Link Scheme in South London. Mental Health Link was developed to help primary and secondary care teams to produce a shared care system based on local needs and resources. The problems it attempts to address are well known and include: duplication of effort, lack of clear roles, acknowledged service gaps, low involvement of primary health care teams in the CPA process, insufficient communication between clinicians, and service users lost to follow-up by both sides.

Mental Health Link was set up to address the needs of adults with severe and long-term mental illnesses, and a pragmatic decision was made to involve only one directorate of the mental health Trust. The two premises underlying the project are: firstly, that individual practices are so different in terms of skills, interests and service user needs that practice-level links are needed; secondly, that care in general practice and at the interface can be significantly improved with minimal resources, and it may be further improved through a shift in resources from secondary to primary care.

The Mental Health Link Scheme is based on the concept that pressure needs to be applied to multiple levers to progress through the stages of formulation, adoption, implementation and maintenance to achieve a successful project. This management strategy is similar to that which uses the SMART approach for short-life working groups (using objectives that are Specific, Measurable, Achievable, Realistic and Timed). In practical terms, the development of Mental Health Link involved collecting evidence on the large number of rarely implemented recommendations from national bodies regarding mental health in primary care. These recommendations were then discussed in the focus groups to establish what managers, doctors and nurses at the grassroots thought about possibilities for change, the obstacles and methods to overcome them. The major themes identified in these focus groups were:

- the difficulty of finding time both to develop services and to see service users
- more involvement was needed for service users' physical health problems
- staff needed support and training, e.g. training for receptionists and nurses
- it was useful to receive advice by telephone/bleep from a psychiatrist
- there was a need for improved communication in the content of letters
- both teams needed improved access by telephone, fax and by-pass numbers
- it was helpful to understand the other team's roles, pressures and limitations
- primary care based practice nurses were prepared to administer medication with support.

By combining this information with ideas from other sources around the country, we concluded that the following practical steps would be necessary to improve joint working at this interface:

- hold joint clinical meetings to discuss difficult service users common to both teams
- establish joint service development meetings, including assessment of current care and needs, planning shared care, and written agreements on service development and training
- share information to improve access, including names and contact details of key members of each team, with direct access telephone numbers and fax numbers
- have better defined roles for primary and secondary services, with case-by-case decisions on who has responsibility for particular service users
- agree shared-care protocols, e.g. on CPA
- agree improved communication, e.g. core information required in referrals, assessments, follow-up and discharge letters

- agree priorities for developing, shared case registers, depots and repeat medication practices, and information systems (for example)
- review staff training needs and agree priorities.

Conclusions

In this chapter we have stressed the following issues. The new context of multiple mental health service purchasers and providers is complex, and it continues to change rapidly. Managers need to ensure that they keep regularly updated on the key operational issues. Much more than in the past, to be effective, NHS managers now need to identify their key partner agencies, to understand how these other agencies differ from their own, to develop close working relationships with their counterparts in those agencies, and to take every appropriate opportunity to collaborate with them. In this way the wide range of mental health services can increasingly operate in a concerted rather than in a fragmented way.

References and further reading

Beeforth, M. and Wood, H. (1996) Purchasing from a user perspective, in G. Thornicroft and G. Strathdee (eds) *Commissioning Mental Health Services*, 205–14. London: HMSO.
Department of Health (1995) *Building Bridges*. London: HMSO.
Department of Health (1997) *The New NHS: Modern, Dependable*. London: HMSO.
Johnson, S., Prossor, D., Bindman, J. and Szmukler, G. (1997) Continuity of care for the severely mentally ill: concepts and measures, *Social Psychiatry and Psychiatric Epidemiology*, 32: 137–42.
Kerwick, S., Tylee, A. and Goldberg, D. (1997) Mental health services in primary care in London, in S. Johnson, R. Ramsay, G. Thornicroft, L. Brooks, P. Lelliot, E. Peck, H. Smith, D. Chisholm, B. Audini, M. Knapp and D. Goldberg (eds) *London's Mental Health*. London: King's Fund.
The NHS and Community Care Act 1990. London: HMSO.
Seymour, E. (1998) *Keys to Engagement*. London: Sainsbury Centre for Mental Health.
Strathdee, G. and Kendrick, A. (1996) *A General Practitioner's Guide to Good Practice in the Care of Individuals with Long-term Mental Health Disorders*. Maudsley Practical Handbook Series, No. 4 (eds G. Strathdee and M. Phelan). London: PRiSM, Institute of Psychiatry.
Thompson, K., Phelan, M., Strathdee, G. and Shiress, D. (1995) *Mental Health Care. A Guide for Housing Workers*. London: Mental Health Foundation.

14 / *Task 6* **Managing the future**

> **Key themes**
>
> In our opinion, trends in the following five areas are likely to domi-
> nate our work in mental health services in the next few years:
>
> - policy
> - organization
> - clinical practice
> - training
> - research.

Introduction

Our intention is that the preceding chapters of this book will have helped to
equip you to face with some equanimity the ongoing challenges of managing mental health services. In this final chapter we shall summarize some
of the key themes that we expect will soon emerge to challenge you further
in future. While all predictions tend to be wrong, at least in retrospect, by
extrapolating the main contemporary trends, we hope that this chapter
will act as an early warning indicator in your preparations to survive the
future!

Policy trends

The likely policy trends in mental health services in the near future are:

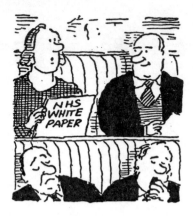

'*I keep getting this
sense of déja vu . . .*'

- the development of primary care groups
- an increasing policy requirement that services command public confidence
- a continuing expectation that capital is raised from the private sector
- new initiatives to counteract prejudice against mental illness
- increasing scrutiny of those registered as disabled
- consultation and research to inform a new mental health Act
- the development of supra-Trust sub-specialist services.

These issues will probably increasingly preoccupy managers in the near future. The need to react to these probable new laws, directives and exhortations will continue to place heavy information loads upon service managers and clinical teams. As yet we see no indication of a slowdown in the publication of new government directives, and so our message is: be prepared!

The creation and influence of primary care groups will add new shape to the contributions of primary care staff to the commissioning of secondary health services. For managers who have not had substantial experience of working with general practice fundholders in recent years, this may require rethinking the way they relate to the primary care level. One example of this influence is that sector team boundaries may in some cases become coterminous with general practice lists or practice boundaries, rather than borough or electoral ward boundaries as is most often the case at present. This may mean, for better or for worse, further reorganization of team boundaries, and will require the negotiation of new service agreements. Further, the current two-dimensional health–social services axis is likely in the future to assume the shape of a triangular or three-dimensional relationship between (i) primary health, (ii) secondary mental health and (iii) social services.

In addition, we expect a revision of the Mental Health Act 1983 or the creation of a new act relevant to the post-institutional era. The Mental Health Act 1983 was strongly influenced by the legal and civil libertarian arguments prominent in the mid-1970s (Gostin 1975). At that time there were about twice today's numbers of psychiatric beds, and the configuration of other services was very different from those now current, with relatively few service users with disabilities supported in the community. We therefore need to recognize how much the wider context has changed. We must now attempt to manage the following balances: (i) the independence and autonomy of service users versus perceived public safety, (ii) the least restrictive alternative versus duty of care to ensure receipt of services, (iii) the duty of professional confidentiality versus multiple service agencies' 'need to know' about clinical information, and (iv) the need to establish traditional medico-legal 'consent' versus newer requirements to assess whether, first, the capacity to give consent is present. All of these dilemmas suggest to us that it is likely that a new mental health Act will soon be necessary.

Organizational trends

We expect that one positive trend will be the increasing practice of integration of mental health and social services with a range of hybrid developments. These newer and sometimes innovative arrangements already include the employment of social services by health providers, and the merging into joint management of health and social services community staff. Examples of this include the integration of needs assessment procedures, the co-location of both teams in shared buildings, the sharing of dedicated mental health merged budgets, and improved planning at middle manager and at chief officer levels. Such arrangements are likely to follow on from the clear demonstration of benefits arising from joint working at the grassroots level.

Other trends at organizational level include:

- an increasingly assertive service user and carer presence
- the growing influence of accreditation procedure – initially discretionary and then mandatory for services
- the introduction of benchmarking standards and inter-organizational comparisons
- the need to comply with a new minimum data set for central returns
- the increasing use of demonstration site dissemination methodologies, e.g. Health Action Zones
- increasing incentives for inter-agency pooling of resources.

One predictable disadvantage of these developments may be that the independent non-medical culture that is often a feature of social services staff – which tends to advocate for service users – may be gradually eroded. For example, in merged teams the social worker may not be sufficiently independent to act as an 'appropriate adult' in relation to the criminal justice system.

Clinical trends

One of the clearest clinical trends at present is the growing expectation that adult mental health services will undertake assessments of the risks posed by service users to themselves or to others. This expectation has emerged relatively rapidly in response to public, and consequently political, concern arising from their focus on the mentally ill as a social threat. There is no strong evidence that the likelihood of being harmed by someone with a mental illness has increased in recent years. Equally, there is no proven association between deinstitutionalization and violence perpetrated by the mentally ill. Nevertheless, the pubic belief in such a connection is now well established, and clinical policy and clinical practice are moving to respond to this change of mood in a remarkably adaptive way.

As yet the scientific value of risk assessments to predict future behaviour (for individual service users) is weak. If current risk assessments were used to identify, for example, those who need medium-secure provision, then they would be likely to indicate that at least ten people should be admitted for every one person who would actually commit a serious assault. This is because our present risk assessment procedures are not very specific, and they tend to over-identify those who are at highest risk of committing violence. Even so, we can expect that risk assessment procedures will soon become a clinically, economically and ethically controversial part of routine adult mental health practice.

Other clinical trends include:

- high-support community homes and hostels
- alternative services to hospital admission
- extension of CMHT hours of operation
- the development of innovative culturally sensitive services
- an increasing focus on the intensity of treatment
- the increasing use of standardized risk assessment procedures
- more use of convergent treatment guidelines and protocols
- more attention to the 'not quite severely mentally ill' groups
- a continuing trend to reduce average length of stay
- newer, more expensive medications to replace older, cheaper ones.

Training trends

One example of the increasing need for team managers to pay attention to staff training is the trend in recent years to employ non-professionally trained community staff to work in the community. These staff offer practical support to people with severe mental illness. Because they are unqualified non-professional workers, the team manager will need to take seriously their training and support needs. Following the NHS and Community Care Act 1990 there has been a rapid increase in the commissioning of this new category of paraprofessional to work directly with service users in their own homes. Community support workers (CSWs) use a variety of approaches including practical help, support, liaison with statutory services and befriending.

As part of the mixed economy brought about by the current community care arrangements, CSWs may be employed by the independent sector as well as by NHS Trusts or social services departments. Some of the reasons for the growth of CSWs are (i) the increasing difficulty of recruiting and retaining professionally trained staff, (ii) the growth of a commissioning culture within social services in particular, and (iii) the stated preferences of service users who value their more informal rapport and down-to-earth practical approach. As a manager you will also need to appreciate the lack of clear lines of professional accountability for this group of staff. Similarly, the absence of national accreditation standards means that tight organizational or contractual accountability arrangements will need to be put in place instead.

Other training trends include:

- training for primary care staff in the detection and treatment of common mental disorders
- training for community mental health staff in cognitive-behavioural treatment and medication compliance
- increasing difficulties recruiting to inner city services
- more use of non-professionally trained direct care staff
- better training on family psycho-educational issues
- an increase in the cultural relevance and sensitivity of service.

Research trends

One of the areas in which we expect – and hope – to see a growth in clinically relevant research is staff burnout. It may not be much of an exaggeration to say that institutions suited staff more than service users, while community facilities suit service users more than staff. Whatever the context, systematic studies of the causes of burnout – now common amongst mental health staff – and its remedies are long overdue. The symptoms of burnout can include unacceptable levels of absenteeism, work-related stress and sickness, and low morale. This is one of the central challenges facing managers, about which there is a deafening silence from the research literature. We see the creation of an evidence base for staff remotivation as a high priority for research and development within the NHS.

Other research trends include:

- more evaluations of 'bread and butter' service components, including in-patient and out-patient care
- crisis cards and advanced directives

- increasing number of effectiveness rather than efficacy studies
- the introduction into routine clinical practice of outcome measures and systematic audit.

To a large extent the future influence of research on clinical practice will depend upon how far research is conducted in ordinary clinical settings. It is important here to keep in mind that efficacy studies measure how far specific interventions achieves their intentions under *ideal, experimental conditions*. More important to managers are effectiveness studies, which are undertaken in routine sites. This trend is likely to accelerate after the establishment of the new National Institute for Clinical Effectiveness.

Managing the future

In the foreseeable future, managers will continue to be central figures within mental health services; they will, however, operate as a new type of manager. Table 14.1 shows some of the ways in which the new role differs from that of the more traditional roles of hospital administrator, or nursing officer, or clinical superintendent. We do not underestimate the extent of these changes, nor the shift of focus that is now required from managers as

Table 14.1 Past and future characteristics of mental health service managers

	Past	*Future*
Base site	institutions	community mental health centre
Habitat	institutions	whole local area
Management line	linear via line managers	via management networks
Orientation	policies and procedures	task orientation. Supplements operational policies with negotiation and persuasion
Style	directive and hierarchical	high profile communicator
Necessary skills	high quality administration	high quality administration
Knowledge base	professional or NHS administrative background	continuing professional management development
Supervision	when possible	essential
Understanding of research	unnecessary	essential
Financial acumen	leave to finance department	vital with delegated budgets
Locus of control	staff control patients	unclear! Staff often feel out of control
Key contacts	departments within the hospital	partner agencies in the locality

a result. This new mould of manager will need: (i) to expect change to be the norm, (ii) to demonstrate high levels of communication skills, and (iii) to work proactively with other agencies across traditional service boundaries.

Within the clinical team, the team leader will need to be supported to develop the range of these management skills relevant to that role, while maintaining clinical expertise. By comparison, more senior managers will need to be fluent in a far wider range of competencies. On the positive side, the scale of the demands facing mental health services are better known now than ever before, the legacy of the formidable institutions is now almost completely eradicated, the voices of users of services are louder and clearer than in any previous time, and the focus on the quality of life that services can help to achieve for service users is now at its sharpest. The coming years will offer the mental health service manager the prospect of unrivalled opportunities to be the critical point of contact between effective clinical treatment and high quality administration.

References and further reading

Department of Health (1997) *The New NHS: Modern and Dependable*. London: HMSO.

Department of Health (1998) *Our Healthier Nation: A Contract for Health*. London: HMSO.

Gostin, L. (1975) *A Human Condition*. London: MIND.

NHS Executive (1996a) *An Audit Pack for Monitoring the Care Programme Approach. Monitoring Tool* (96): 16, HSG(96)/LASSL. Leeds: Department of Health.

NHS Executive (1996b) *24 Hour Nursed Care for People with Severe and Enduring Mental Illness*. Leeds: Department of Health.

NHS Executive (1996c) *Spectrum of Care. Local Services for People with Mental Health Problems*. London: Department of Health.

Index

REALLY MANAGING HEALTH CARE

Valerie Iles

More and more health care professionals are being asked to take on managerial responsibilities. At the same time the pressure on people and resources increases unremittingly and the need for good management increases with it.

Really Managing Health Care draws a distinction between traditional management in health care and real management, arguing that the former concentrates on activities which are complicated but easy whereas the latter requires a commitment to principles which are simple but hard. It introduces health care professionals to a wide range of basic management concepts and demonstrates their application within health care.

Really Managing Health Care is written specifically for people suspicious of management jargon. It proposes that all health professionals have an interest in developing their skills in real management; and that in doing so they will enhance their clinical skills. It explores the parallels between good clinical and good managerial practice and suggests that clinical effectiveness suffers wherever the principles of real management are not adopted throughout the health care organization. Failure to observe these principles, the author argues, is as evident at the top of these organizations as anywhere else.

Contents
Introduction – Really managing people: working through others – Really managing people: working with others – Really managing people: working for others – Really managing change – Really managing money – Really managing yourself – Really managing organizations – Case studies – Conclusions – Notes.

208pp   0 335 19414 1 (Paperback)   0 335 19415 X (Hardback)

PURCHASING FOR HEALTH
A MULTIDISCIPLINARY INTRODUCTION TO THE THEORY AND PRACTICE OF HEALTH PURCHASING

John Øvretveit

Health purchasing has grown in prominence as a result of health reform in Europe and the USA to become one of the world's biggest industries. People's health increasingly depends on the skills and abilities of health purchasing managers, yet little is known about the subject. Ordinary people are becoming aware of the sums spent in their name by 'faceless bureaucrats', and cannot see what value health purchasers add. Although health purchasing is more than paying bills and contracting services, there is uncertainty about the purpose and future role of purchasing organizations in different health systems.

This first book on the subject views health purchasing – both public and private – as a service industry. It argues that, to survive, purchasers have to be more than agents of cost control and must win public support by shaping technological and service changes to uphold our rights and interests. Purchasers need to use service management methods and organization to improve their services to ordinary people.

This book contributes to the theory and practice of the new management discipline of health purchasing, and to an understanding of health purchasing organizations, both public and private. It examines the purpose and methods of health purchasing as a service industry in a rapidly changing and unique type of market. Although concentrating on public health purchasing in the British National Health Service, the book does so in a way which allows comparisons to be made with purchasing in other countries. It presents practical approaches, concepts and models which have helped purchasing managers and governing board members to tackle key issues. It draws on experience from a variety of sources including a development programme for seven integrated NHS purchasing agencies and the author's research into health reforms in Europe and the USA.

Contents
Purchasing for health – Purchasing and 'market reform' – Health commissioning: purpose and work – 'Decentralized' or 'locality' purchasing – Justifiable purchasing: rationing, priorities, effectiveness and outcome – Contracting and contracts – Quality in purchasing – Collaboration with local authorities – Developing primary and community health services – Purchasing primary health care and the role of the FHSA – Integrating primary and secondary health purchasing – Purchasing agency organization – The future for health purchasing: financing, competition and values – References – Bibliography – Index.

368pp   0 335 19332 3 (Paperback)   0 335 19333 1 (Hardback)

DOCTORS AND MANAGEMENT IN THE NATIONAL HEALTH SERVICE

Gordon Marnoch

This book presents an assessment of the impact of public services management reform on doctors working in the National Health Service and examines the emergent possibilities for harnessing doctors' skills in the management processes of the future. Issues of organizational change, the development of medical managers and the use of performance management techniques are critically examined. Recent developments in the United States are used to provide a sense of perspective on the contemporary relationship which doctors working in the NHS have with its management processes.

While the book will be used on a range of undergraduate and postgraduate courses in management and social sciences the contents will be of particular interest to doctors and medical students.

Contents
Acknowledgements – Introduction: the management agenda for doctors – The pre-history of contemporary medical management in the National Health Service – Doctors and the market reforms – The medical managers – Doctors and performance management in the National Health Service – Fit for purpose?: organization and medical management – Doctors and health service management: reinventing the relationship? – References – Index.

144pp   0 335 19344 7 (Paperback)   0 335 19345 5 (Hardback)